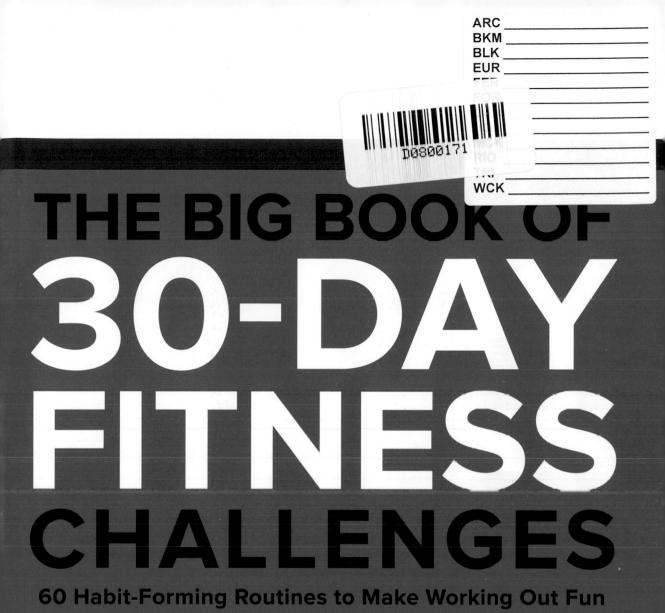

THE BIG BOOK OF
30-DAY
FITNESS
CHALLENGES

60 Habit-Forming Routines to Make Working Out Fun

ANDIE THUESON

Published in the U.S. by:
Ulysses Press
P.O. Box 3440
Berkeley, CA 94703
www.ulyssespress.com

ISBN: 978-1-61243-934-1
Library of Congress Control Number: 2019905572

Printed in the United States by Versa Press
10 9 8 7 6 5 4 3 2 1

Acquisitions editor: Bridget Thoreson
Managing editor: Claire Chun
Editor: Lauren Harrison
Proofreader: Renee Rutledge
Front cover design: Rebecca Lown
Interior design and layout: what!design @ whatweb.com
Artwork from Shutterstock.com: cover exercise equipment © snorks; cover stick figures © SoleilC; pages 6, 8, 12, 19, 22, 26, 28, 31, 36, 62, 69, 71, 77, 89, 94, 120 © NotionPic; pages 10, 97, 104, 117 © Igogosha; page 15 © Dmytro Bochkov; pages 16, 33, 35, 66, 86, 87 © SunshineVector; pages 20, 21, 111, 114 (woman) © Macrovector; pages 25, 73, 75, 78, 82 © solar22; pages 38–39, 109 © pikepicture; pages 47, 118 © Studio_G; pages 65, 106, 114 © ONYXprj; page 85 © Nadya_Art; page 90 © Artisticco; page 93 © Mountain Brothers; page 98 © VolkovaAnna; page 101 © Leyasw; page 102 © Ciripasca; page 112 © tynyuk; page 123 © Toltemara; page 124 © AmazeinDesign; pages 126–27 © AnastasiaSonne

CONTENTS

FLEXIBILITY

FOOD

SELF-CARE

CLEAR HEAD, CLEAR HEART

APPENDIX

ABOUT THE AUTHOR

INTRODUCTION

In my life, I have lived and learned a lot along the way. After having my first baby, I remember being overcome with postpartum depression. I had this tiny infant that needed me constantly, and I was exhausted. I felt overwhelmed and completely lost. My life was spinning out of control and I couldn't find a point of reference that would ground me.

At that time, I learned the power of goals. I learned that you absolutely can change the trajectory of your life in 30 days.

Goals, however, can get a bad rap. We typically write out these goals at the beginning of the year in the form of resolutions that are filled with optimism and hope. We hope that this time will be different, this time we will make changes that stick.

But our goals can easily lose their luster and gleam as reality sets in and we lose momentum. Next thing we know, it's mid-February and we're right back where we started.

And yet, I am a firm believer in goals. If you don't have *any* goals, you'll find yourself sleepwalking through life. But how do we make goals stick?

Here's something that has helped me, and I hope that it will help you as well: **Stop waiting for a start date!** *Stop* **assigning your goals to a certain date.**

Whether it's a Monday or a Friday, choose to make your goals a priority. Choose to start every day with a plan. There is a power in today! Not tomorrow or two weeks from now—today. Start with one day, then two, then a week, and you'll be amazed by how much you can change your life in just 30 days.

As you flip through these 60 challenges, you might feel overwhelmed. So many options, so many challenges to embrace and try. The trick is to just pick one challenge at a time. Give yourself grace; you will not complete every day perfectly, and that is okay. Keep dusting yourself off, keep picking up this book, and try again!

Every day is a gift. Every day you can choose to change your life and become a healthier, happier, and more positive version of yourself. Spoiler alert: I know you can do this!

With love and gratitude, Andie Thueson

1. RUN A COUCH TO 5K

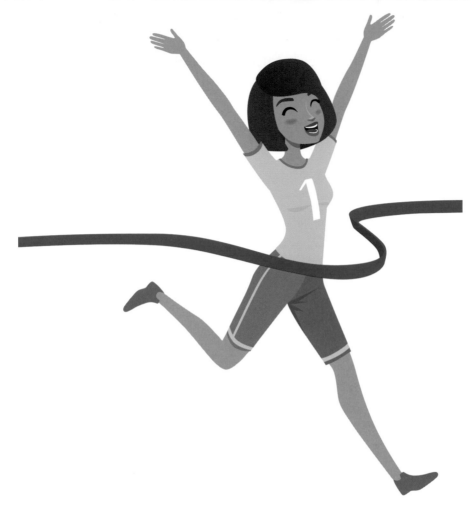

I used to tell people that if they ever saw me running down the street it was either because I stole something or someone was chasing me—either way, they had better call the cops. But after having my second baby, I decided it was time to branch out and give this crazy "running thing" a try. It couldn't be that bad, right?! People seemed to sign up to run in races all the time, just for fun. Maybe I was missing something.

So I decided I would join some friends and sign up for a local 5k before even running my first mile. After I committed to the race, I found a great Couch to 5k outline online and started mentally preparing to leave all my friends in the literal and proverbial dust.

During my first practice run I remember hitting, maybe, 500 yards and I was wheezing and thinking, "So this is how it all ends." I thought I was literally dying! But as I continued to train, I began to look forward to my runs. What was once something I dreaded and only did because I had committed began to be one of the best parts of my day.

Over the years I have continued to run and train for all kinds of races. I have done half marathons, 10ks, and even 24-hour crazy-hard relay races. But I think my biggest sense of accomplishment came from when I completed that first 5k! The time is now to make your move. Running will empower you and give you a great sense of self-worth. You are amazing and you *can* do it!

Day 1:	Run 10 minutes, walk 1 minute, repeat 2 times
Day 2:	Rest or cross-train
Day 3:	Run 12 minutes, walk 1 minute, repeat 2 times
Day 4:	Rest
Day 5:	Run 13 minutes, walk 1 minute, repeat 2 times
Day 6:	Rest or cross-train
Day 7:	Rest
Day 8:	Run 15 minutes, walk 1 minute, repeat 2 times
Day 9:	Rest or cross-train
Day 10:	Run 17 minutes, walk 1 minute, run 7 minutes
Day 11:	Rest
Day 12:	Run 19 minutes, walk 1 minute, run 7 minutes
Day 13:	Rest or cross-train
Day 14:	Rest
Day 15:	Run 20 minutes, walk 1 minute, run 6 minutes
Day 16:	Rest or cross-train
Day 17:	Run 24 minutes
Day 18:	Rest
Day 19:	Run 26 minutes
Day 20:	Rest or cross-train
Day 21:	Rest
Day 22:	Run 28 minutes
Day 23:	Rest or cross-train
Day 24:	Run 30 minutes
Day 25:	Rest
Day 26:	Run 20 minutes
Day 27:	Rest
Day 28:	Run 25 minutes
Day 29:	Rest
Day 30:	Race day—run 5k (3.1 miles)!

2. MAKE THOSE KIDS MOVE MORE (OR MOVE LIKE A KID!)

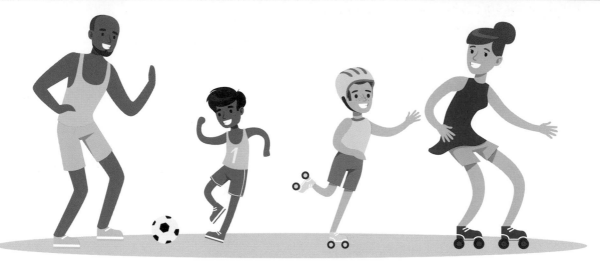

Growing up, I remember leaving my house at the crack of dawn to meet the neighborhood kids to play. We would run and laugh, breezing through each other's houses to grab a snack, and then it was right back outside for more fun! I played until the streetlamps would flicker on and then headed home satisfied after a long day of fun.

Not to sound like a grouchy old grandma, but man, kids these days! I have to set timers on my kids' devices to remind them that there are other things in this world besides TV, *Minecraft*, and *Fortnite*. Am I alone in this? Maybe your kids love heading outside, playing and riding bikes all day, and if so, you're doing awesome! But if you're like me and need some ideas on how exactly one gets said kids off the couch, then stick with me.

Being active is vital to your children's health and well-being. According to KidsHealth.org, studies have shown that exercise builds strong muscles and bones, helps control weight, decreases the risk of developing type 2 diabetes, improves sleep, and helps children have a better outlook on life.

To help promote a healthy and fit lifestyle for kids and to help my own children find ways to free their eyes from screens, I've rounded up 50 ways to get your kids moving and active. Active kids are healthier kids, so make a goal and commit to squeezing in time for one of these activities every day for 30 days. Bonus points if you complete it with them!

1. **Hopscotch**
2. **Four Square**
3. ***Phineas and Ferb* Workout—kids love this one because screen time!**

(go to www.maybeiwill.com/ challengesbook for how to do this)
4. **Kickball**
5. **Tennis**

6. **Swings**

7. **Take 10,000 Steps a Day challenge on page 16**

8. **Basketball—play a simple game of HORSE or PIG**

9. **Ring around the Rosie—perfect for littles**

10. **Simon Says**

11. **Red Rover**

12. **Bike ride**

13. **Take an after-dinner walk and play I Spy**

14. **Soccer**

15. **Tag**

16. **Take it to the curb for step-ups**

17. **Do a Marathon in a Month on page 10**

18. **T-ball**

19. **Tetherball**

20. **Hula-hoop—make it a game and see who can keep going the longest**

21. **Jump rope**

22. **Make an obstacle course**

23. **Go for a hike**

24. **Race!**

25. **Whiffle ball**

26. **Frisbee**

27. **Miniature golf**

28. **Plan a scavenger hunt**

29. **Plant a garden**

30. **Jump on a trampoline**

31. **Roller-skate or rollerblade**

32. **Swim**

33. **Handstand contest**

34. **Geocache (see Geocaching.com)**

35. **Climb trees—make sure the trees are sturdy**

36. **Water balloon volleyball—pass water balloons over the net with bedsheets**

37. **Tug-of-war**

38. **Toss the football around**

39. **Two-legged races**

40. **Egg-walk relays—who can keep the egg whole?**

41. **Indoor rock climbing**

42. **Grab a sled or some skis and enjoy the snow**

43. **Dance party—nothing beats an impromptu dance-a-thon**

44. **Have your kids lead you in a workout**

45. **Set up a Slip 'N Slide**

46. **Run through the sprinklers**

47. **Duck Duck Goose**

48. **Take a walk and play Don't Step on the Crack**

49. **Hit the park and cook up a workout, or just play!**

50. **Take Twister outdoors**

3. DO A MARATHON IN A MONTH

The idea of this challenge is for you as a family to log 26.2 miles overall for 30 days. Each day you will count the number of miles completed, keeping track so that you hit 26.2 miles by the end of the month.

Does that mean you have to actually run all 26.2 miles? No! There are so many fun and creative ways to get your miles in:

Biking: Family bike rides are a great option!

Hiking: I love using the free app AllTrails to help find family-friendly trails nearby.

Running: Maybe not the full 26.2, but a nice little jog around the neighborhood can be a great way to log some of those miles.

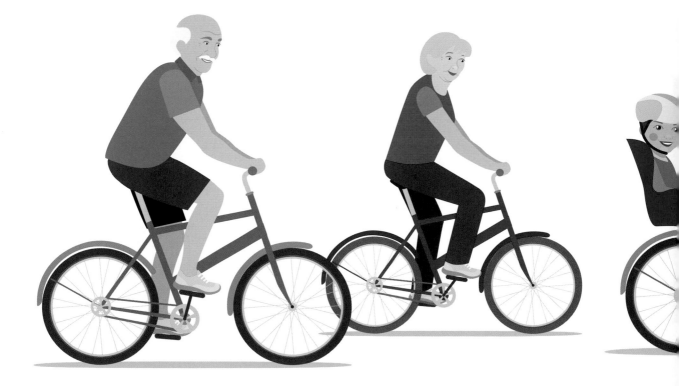

| **Skating:** | Dust off those blades or skates and get rolling! |
| **Walking:** | Even if you have super little ones, throw them in the stroller and the challenge can still be completed. |

These are all fantastic ways to get exercise, and mixing it up is a fun way to get the whole family on board.

Just think how proud your kids will feel when they say they completed a marathon! During the summer months or when nice weather permits, they can do a marathon a month all summer long.

Be creative, have fun, and get those miles in. Healthy kids are happy kids!

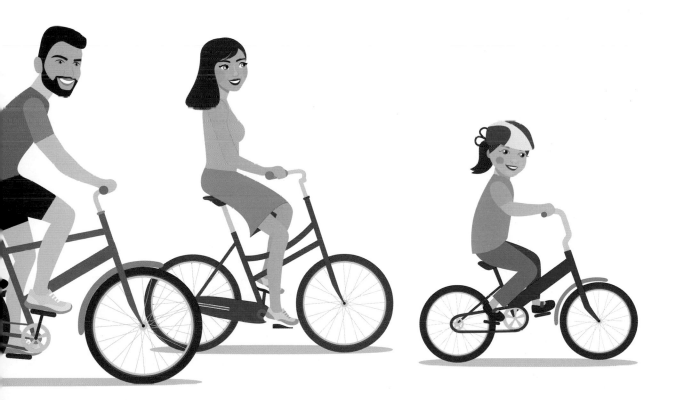

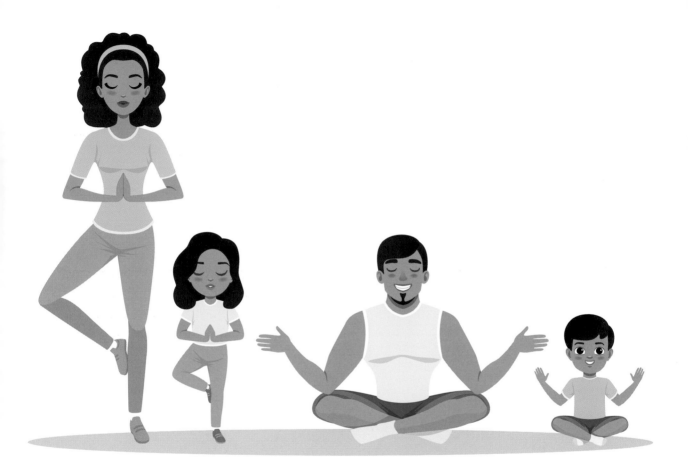

This challenge is for those who find themselves terrified to start working out or feel like they are out of shape and have no idea where to start. For the next 30 days, all you need to do is move for 5 minutes! That's it. This super-simple challenge will help you to get in the habit of moving a little bit each day and hopefully give you a boost of confidence to start adding more and more time.

We are all crazy busy, but hey, everyone can squeeze in 5 minutes!

If you don't know how to do an exercise, go to www.maybeiwill.com/challengesbook for instructions.

Here are 30 activities you can do for 5 minutes at a time. Go in order, mix it up, or pick and choose your favorites.

1. Walk
2. Tippy toes—Rock back and forth on your toes and every so often hold the "up" for a couple seconds.
3. Bike ride
4. Arm circles
5. Frisbee
6. Leg lifts
7. Dance
8. Air punches
9. Biceps curls
10. Jump rope
11. Windmills
12. Cherry pickers
13. Jumping jacks
14. Squats
15. Lunges
16. Basketball
17. Trunk twists
18. Push-ups
19. Play tag
20. Vacuum
21. Pull weeds
22. Yoga
23. Leg kicks
24. Chair rolls—If you work in an office, this is a great one. Move your rolling chair around using the strength of your legs.
25. Dust
26. Step-outs—Using a resistance band carefully placed around your mid-thighs, lower to a squat and step out. Take five steps to the right and then five steps to the left. Keep it going for 5 minutes.
27. Curb or stair steps
28. Swim
29. T raises
30. Triceps dips

5. WORK OUT WITH YOUR BODY WEIGHT

When it comes to fitness, there are a few key moves that you could use to build a stronger, healthier body, even if they were the only things you did. Body weight exercises are amazing and a fantastic resource if you are low on time and don't have access to a gym. If you don't know how to do an exercise, go to www.maybeiwill.com/challengesbook for instructions.

So if you want to challenge yourself and push yourself a little bit more each day without the need for a fancy gym membership or equipment, this simple challenge is right up your alley.

SQUATS—Will help to tone your legs and, of course, that tush! Some variations to try over the next 30 days:

- → **Plie Squats**
- → **Sumo Squats**
- → **Prison Squats**
- → **Basic Squats**
- → **Squat Pulses**
- → **Squat Jumps**
- → **Wall Squats**

LUNGES—They don't get quite the glory of squats, but these lovelies are great for toning your whole leg. Some variations to try:

- → **Front Lunges**
- → **Reverse Lunges**
- → **Side Lunges**
- → **Walking Lunges**
- → **Curtsy Lunge**
- → **Clock Lunges**

SIT-UPS—These may seem pretty basic, but they're great for building a strong core. If you need some extra help, you can sneak your toes under a couch until you can manage without using the couch.

PUSH-UPS—In my humble opinion, these are one of the best overall exercises that pretty much targets everything. Start with modified push-ups if needed, from your knees or supported by a wall or other surface, working up to do one or two on your toes, and then keep challenging yourself to do more and more full push-ups. You may surprise yourself!

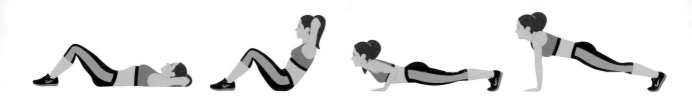

Day 1:	10 Squats, 5 Sit-Ups	Day 16:	50 Lunges, 20 Push-Ups
Day 2:	10 Lunges, 5 Push-Ups	Day 17:	55 Squats, 22 Sit-Ups
Day 3:	20 Squats	Day 18:	55 Lunges, 22 Push-Ups
Day 4:	20 Lunges, 10 Sit-Ups	Day 19:	60 Squats, 24 Sit-Ups
Day 5:	25 Squats, 10 Push-Ups	Day 20:	60 Lunges, 24 Push-Ups
Day 6:	25 Lunges	Day 21:	65 Squats, 26 Sit-Ups
Day 7:	30 Squats, 12 Sit-Ups	Day 22:	65 Lunges, 26 Push-Ups
Day 8:	30 Lunges, 12 Push-Ups	Day 23:	70 Squats, 28 Sit-Ups
Day 9:	35 Squats, 14 Sit-Ups	Day 24:	70 Lunges, 28 Push-Ups
Day 10:	35 Lunges, 14 Sit-Ups	Day 25:	75 Squats, 30 Sit-Ups
Day 11:	40 Squats, 16 Sit-Ups	Day 26:	75 Lunges, 30 Push-Ups
Day 12:	40 Lunges, 16 Push-Ups	Day 27:	80 Squats, 32 Sit-Ups
Day 13:	45 Squats, 18 Sit-Ups	Day 28:	80 Lunges, 32 Push-Ups
Day 14:	45 Lunges, 18 Push-Ups	Day 29:	85 Squats, 35 Sit-Ups
Day 15:	50 Squats, 20 Sit-Ups	Day 30:	85 Lunges, 35 Push-Ups

By the end of 30 days, you'll be amazed that you can do 85 squats, 85 lunges, 35 sit-ups, and 35 push-ups. I know you can do it!

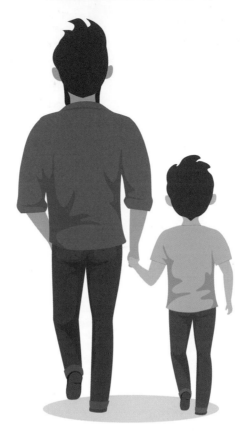

Fitness trackers have become quite the rage and can be a great way to help push you and challenge you to stay more active throughout the day. For this 30-day challenge your aim will be to successfully get in 10,000 steps a day for the full month.

When I first set that as my daily goal, I thought it would be a piece of cake, but quickly realized that 10,000 steps are a lot, especially when I'm home all day. But getting more steps in the day is a great way for fitness beginners to get started or add a little extra exercise no matter what level of fitness you may be at currently.

On average, taking 10,000 steps daily will burn between 400 and 500 calories. Here are 25 ways to get stepping more (for more ideas, see Compete for Your Daily Steps, page 18):

1. **When grocery shopping, make extra trips around the perimeter of the store.**

2. **Pace while you brush your teeth.**

3. **Use the restroom upstairs or downstairs instead of the one closest to you.**

4. Walk around the block while your child is at their lessons.

5. Pace the room when you are waiting, like at the doctor, dentist, or airport.

6. Park far away from your destination instead of fighting for that primo spot.

7. Before you head outside to check the mail, take a lap around your entire house.

8. Walk to the store if you're picking up only a couple items that are easily tote-able.

9. Always pace when talking on the phone. I do laps around my dining room table.

10. Walk your kid to school instead of fighting the carpool line.

11. Headed to a mall? Mall-walking is a great way to get some serious window shopping and major steps in at the same time.

12. Set a timer to get up every half-hour or so and walk around.

13. Instead of making your kids get stuff for you (guilty!), get things for yourself!

14. Just say no to escalators and elevators—make it a life choice to always take the stairs.

15. If you have to visit two stores that are relatively close together, park midway between the two and walk to both.

16. Make an after-dinner stroll with the family a daily habit.

17. On date night, always include a leisurely walk around the area where the restaurant is.

18. Instead of playing "pack mule" with the grocery bags, take them in from the car one at a time.

19. Empty each dish one at a time from the dishwasher, putting them away before grabbing the next.

20. Play hide-and-seek with your kids.

21. Instead of fast-forwarding during commercials on recorded TV programs, get up and pace during that time.

22. Mow the lawn.

23. Walk your kids to the park and then walk laps around the perimeter.

24. When you put your clothes away, do it one item at a time.

25. Pace when folding laundry.

Don't think you have to do all 10,000 steps in one big chunk. Just break it up and keep moving. Every time you make the effort to get a few more steps in, it will make a difference. Here's to 30 days of getting a little bit healthier one extra step at a time.

7. COMPETE FOR YOUR DAILY STEPS

This challenge is great for a group and is an amazing way for your friends, family, or office team (to name a few groups) to be more active and get in on the fun! You'll need pedometers or activity trackers for all participants. Inexpensive pedometers are everywhere these days, and I have even found some at our local dollar store, so no need to spend lots of extra money on this one.

Once members have received their trackers, it's time to get walking! You might be amazed to see exactly how many steps your kids take every day.

At the end of the night right before bed, record everyone's steps for the day. My family uses a chalkboard in our kitchen. It makes it fun to see who is in the lead and how many more steps you need to take to pass them.

Whoever has the most steps at the end of 30 days is the winner!

IDEAS FOR PRIZES:

» Winner gets to pick where the family goes out to dinner

» Winner gets to have others do their chores for a week

» Winner gets to pick what's for dinner for a week

» Winner gets a personally decorated trophy from a thrift store

» Winner gets a gift card from their favorite store

Sometimes getting in extra steps can be tricky, so here are 25 ways to up your daily step totals (for more ideas, see Take 10,000 Steps a Day, page 16):

1. **Vacuum more often (my house definitely needs it!)**

2. **Walk to the gym.**

3. **Go for an early-morning walk around the neighborhood.**

4. **Play tag with your kids.**

5. **Pace when cooking.**

6. **Don't go to bed unless you've met your goal—take laps around the room to get it in. Get your significant other involved.**

7. **Walk in place in the shower. Just don't slip!**

8. **Get your dance on—turn the music on and it's an instant dance party.**

9. **If it's less than a mile, choose to walk.**

10. Before I make myself a snack, I walk our stairs twice.

11. Walk while typing an email.

12. If you're on Facebook, Instagram, or Twitter while on your phone, pace!

13. Walk your house, following the floorboard line throughout your entire place.

14. Play Duck-Duck-Goose with your kids.

15. For every time your kids say, "I'm bored," they have to lap the neighborhood with you.

16. Go hiking.

17. Go to your local high school and walk the track (if it's less than a mile, walk there too!).

18. Always return your shopping cart to the cart return one aisle over.

19. March in place.

20. Put some spunk in your step—the more you mosey and move while walking, the more calories you burn.

21. Do an evening clean sweep. Walk your house and put away stuff that needs putting away, one item at a time.

22. Walk to visit a friend. I'm sure your stopping by will brighten their day!

23. Explore your neighborhood on foot. Check out different routes and walking paths if you have them.

24. If you work, instead of messaging someone, get up and walk to their desk.

25. Put the remote down and walk to change the channel or adjust the volume.

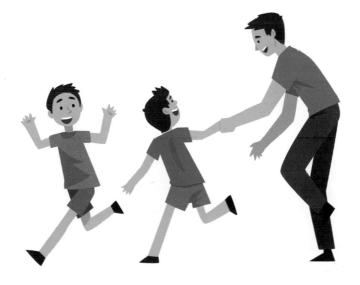

8. WORK OUT WITH A DECK OF CARDS

For this challenge, you'll need a deck of cards and some light weights. To prepare, clear the deck of all cards below the number five. So get rid of all the 2s, 3s, and 4s—no cheating!

If you don't know how to do an exercise, go to www.maybeiwill.com/challengesbook for instructions.

Every day, shuffle the deck and pick four cards. Lay them face down in front of you. The suit of each card will determine what exercises you'll be doing that day:

Spade:	Jumping Jacks
Club:	Biceps Curls
Diamond:	Squats
Heart:	Skaters
Joker:	Push-Ups

The number on each card will determine how many repetitions of each exercise you'll do.

If you flip a Jack, Queen, or King, that equals 10 reps. An Ace is 11 reps and a Joker is 12 reps.

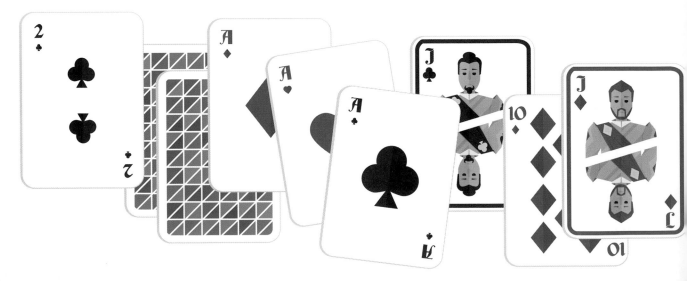

Let's look at an example:

CARDS FLIPPED:

→ **5 of Hearts**

→ **9 of Clubs**

→ **1 Joker**

→ **Ace of Spades**

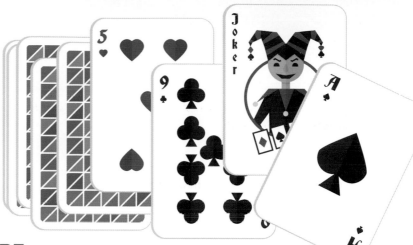

WORKOUT WOULD BE:

→ **5 Skaters (do one on each side to complete one full repetition)**

→ **9 Biceps Curls (do one on each side to complete one full repetition)**

→ **12 Push-Ups**

→ **11 Jumping Jacks**

Beginner level: Complete 1 to 2 sets

Moderate level: Complete 3 to 5 sets

Advanced level: Complete 5 or more times

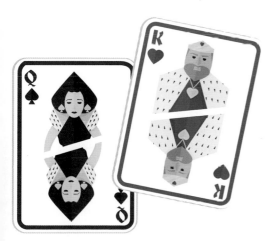

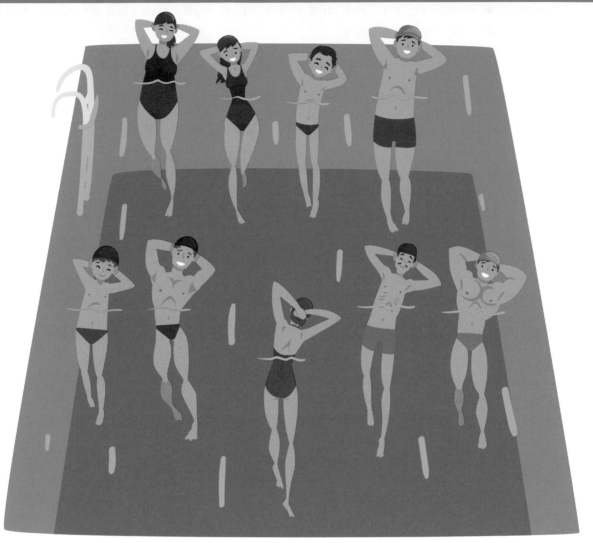

For many of us, finding our perfect workout can be tough. But I believe that if you find a mode of exercise that you truly love, you will never struggle getting yourself to class or to the gym. There are so many awesome resources out there both online and within your own community. So for the next 30 days, I want you to try new workouts and find *your* thing. Give the following exercises a go, and hopefully on the other side of 30 days you will have found your fitness soulmate.

Do all these classes and modes of exercise or try a handful—the idea is just to get out there and try new things. But most of all, have fun! Exercise and fitness should be a celebration of what our bodies are capable of, not a punishment for something we have eaten.

Some fun things to remember: Most studios offer a free trial class so that you can test things out and see if you like it. There is also ClassPass, a service that lets you try many different classes at different studios for one fixed monthly price. And let's not forget the power of YouTube and the internet—you can find many of these workouts online for free.

Day 1:	Yoga	**Day 17:**	Swimming
Day 2:	Spin	**Day 18:**	Hot yoga
Day 3:	Zumba	**Day 19:**	Circuit training
Day 4:	Boxing	**Day 20:**	Pound fitness
Day 5:	Dance	**Day 21:**	High fitness
Day 6:	Martial arts	**Day 22:**	Go for a hike
Day 7:	Go for a run	**Day 23:**	Tennis
Day 8:	CrossFit	**Day 24:**	Hip-hop dance
Day 9:	Pilates	**Day 25:**	Water aerobics
Day 10:	Tabata workout	**Day 26:**	Body Pump
Day 11:	Kickboxing	**Day 27:**	TRX
Day 12:	HIIT workout (see page 24)	**Day 28:**	Aerial yoga
Day 13:	Boot camp	**Day 29:**	Rowing
Day 14:	Weight training	**Day 30:**	Group fitness class of choice—look what your local gym offers and try something I haven't even thought to list!
Day 15:	Barre fitness		
Day 16:	Power walking		

10. JUST DO HIIT!

What is HIIT? It stands for "high-intensity interval training." And believe it or not, creating your own HIIT workout is super-easy.

Start with a light 5-minute warm-up. This can be a nice walk, jogging in place, yoga stretches—just loosen up your muscles.

Next you will alternate between 1 minute of high-intensity strength exercises and 2 minutes of medium-intensity cardio. Take a 30-second rest between each cycle.

If you don't know how to do an exercise, go to www.maybeiwill.com/challengesbook for instructions.

SO EACH ROUND WILL LOOK LIKE THIS:

» 1 minute high-intensity strength exercises

» 2 minutes medium-intensity cardio

» 30 seconds rest

» Repeat as many times as you would like, ideally for 20 to 30 total rounds.

CHOOSE A HIGH-INTENSITY STRENGTH EXERCISE:

→ **Push-Ups**

→ **Triceps Dips**

→ **Planks**

→ **Side Planks**

→ **Hip Drop Planks**

→ **Overhead Presses**

→ **Biceps Curls**

→ **Chest Flies**

→ **Chest Presses**

→ **Renegade Rows**

→ **Bent-Over Rows**

→ **Mason Twists**

→ **Criss Crosses**

→ **Squats**

→ **Sumo Squats**

→ **Side Lunges**

→ **Curtsy Lunges**

→ **Reverse Lunges**

→ **Glute Bridges**

→ **Step-Ups**

→ **Wall Sits**

→ **Deadlifts**

CHOOSE A MEDIUM-INTENSITY CARDIO EXERCISE:

- → **Burpees**
- → **Jumping Jacks**
- → **High Knees**
- → **Heismans**
- → **Ladders**
- → **Mountain Climbers**
- → **Jogging in Place**
- → **Jump Rope**

- → **Skaters**
- → **Inch Worms**
- → **Surrenders**
- → **Kickboxing Kicks**
- → **Four Corners**
- → **Jump Squats**
- → **Jumping Lunges**

NOW LET'S PLAN OUT YOUR 30 DAYS:

Days 1–6:	10 to 15 minutes HIIT workout
Day 7:	Rest
Days 8–13:	15 to 20 minutes HIIT workout
Day 14:	Rest
Days 15–20:	20 to 25 minutes HIIT workout
Day 21:	Rest
Days 22–27:	25 to 30 minutes HIIT workout
Day 28:	Rest
Days 29–30:	30 minutes HIIT workout

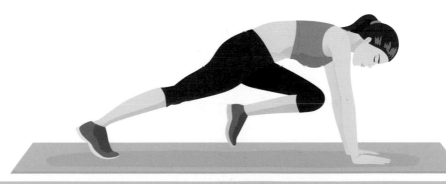

11. TAKE THE COUPLES FITNESS CHALLENGE

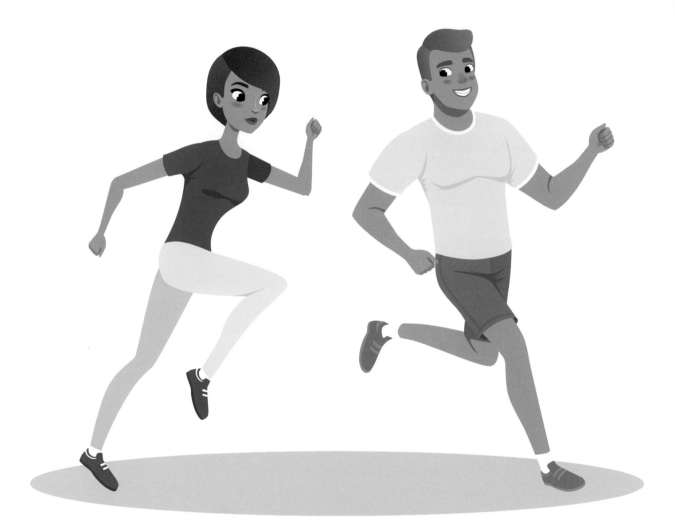

Let's face it, we humans hate to lose. That's why a little friendly competition is a very effective way to stay on track when you want to lose weight.

This challenge is designed to help you create healthy habits with a little friendly competition. So grab your spouse, partner, friend, coworker, or other human you'd like to challenge, and let's do this!

POINTS WILL BE AWARDED FOR THE FOLLOWING:

» 5 points for working out for at least 30 minutes

» 1 point for every 8 ounces of water consumed

» 5 points for going all day without processed sugar

» 1 point for every mile you run or jog

» 5 points for 4 rounds of abs exercises, 20 reps each

» 5 points for meeting or staying under your caloric goal for the day

» 10 bonus points for doing 20 minutes of extra physical activity. This can be a walk after dinner, a bike ride with the kids, or anything that gets you moving.

POINTS WILL BE LOST FOR THE FOLLOWING:

» Lose 5 points for drinking soda

» Lose 5 points for eating fast food

Keep track of your daily points and then add them up at the end to declare the winner!

At our house, we like to put a little extra skin in the game and make friendly wagers. Hate to fold laundry? Make the loser do it! Or how about a relaxing massage for the winner? Have fun with it and be creative.

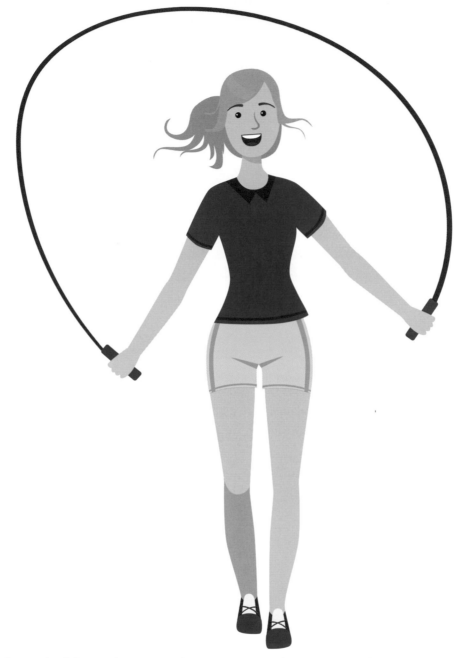

A couple of years back I started going to a boxing gym to work out. Every so often "jumping rope for 5 minutes" would be scribbled across the board and I would inwardly curse its existence.

You see, I hated jumping rope.

But there it was staring me in the face, so I would give it a go and try my best. I struggled hard at first! I would have to take all kinds of breaks which was so crazy to me because I was in pretty good shape. But jumping rope is a completely different form of exercise than what I had been doing. It took some time to build up my endurance.

Jumping rope is an extremely effective form of exercise. You can burn 15 to 20 calories a minute! Just a 5-minute session can burn 100 calories.

For the next 30 days, work up to 5 minutes of jumping rope:

Day 1:	30 seconds	**Day 16:**	2½ minutes
Day 2:	30 seconds	**Day 17:**	3 minutes
Day 3:	1 minute	**Day 18:**	3 minutes
Day 4:	1 minute	**Day 19:**	3 minutes
Day 5:	1 minute	**Day 20:**	3 minutes
Day 6:	1 minute	**Day 21:**	3 minutes
Day 7:	1 minute	**Day 22:**	4 minutes
Day 8:	90 seconds	**Day 23:**	4 minutes
Day 9:	90 seconds	**Day 24:**	4 minutes
Day 10:	2 minutes	**Day 25:**	4 minutes
Day 11:	2 minutes	**Day 26:**	4 minutes
Day 12:	2 minutes	**Day 27:**	5 minutes
Day 13:	2 minutes	**Day 28:**	5 minutes
Day 14:	2 minutes	**Day 29:**	5 minutes
Day 15:	2½ minutes	**Day 30:**	5 minutes

This challenge is a great way to squeeze in a very effective workout in a super-short amount of time. If you struggle to find time to work out, this is a great challenge to tackle!

13. TAKE THE STAIRS

I think one of the easiest and quickest ways to add some extra fitness into our days is to embrace the power of stairs. They are those nasty little buggers we tend to avoid like the plague because they leave us winded, but stairs are a very effective way to burn calories and shape and tone your booty and legs.

So for the next 30 days, stairs are your new bestie. Elevators and escalators no longer exist in your world—only stairs.

If you're like me and work from home, the stairs in your house may be the only ones you encounter. Here's a quick and effective stair workout you can try on those days, where "taking the stairs" is not an option:

→ **Run up and down your stairs as fast as you can for 45 seconds.**

→ **Then take a 1-minute walking break.**

→ **Repeat 8 to 10 times.**

→ **You can start with 15 to 20 seconds of running your stairs and build up to 45 seconds.**

→ **If you live in a home without stairs, you'll have to be a little more proactive. Most high schools have great stadiums that are perfect for stair runs.**

→ **Or head to the gym and use the stair machine for a bit. Start with 5 minutes and work your way up to 20 minutes, increasing your intensity a bit each time.**

→ **Go master those stairs and you will become the stair master!**

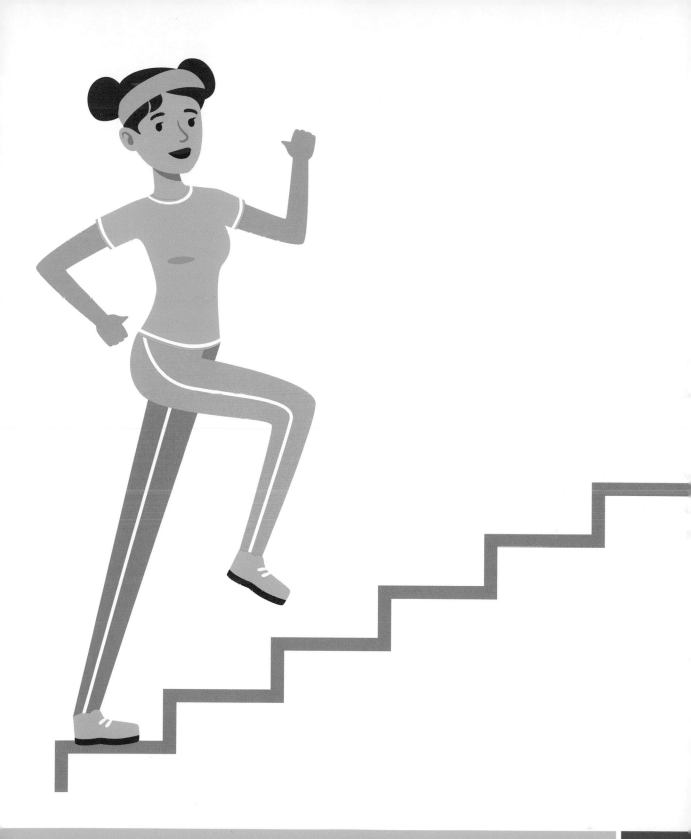

14. TAKE A HIKE

One of my greatest joys in life is hiking. There is something that I absolutely adore about being in the mountains and exploring. Whether you live near the mountains or not, there is always a cool path to discover. During the week (when it is harder and you have less time to head to the mountains to hike), you can enjoy a nature walk in a local park or your neighborhood. Get creative and find places that make it easier to head outside and bask in nature.

For the next 30 days choose to get out and explore!

→ **One amazing tool that I use frequently is the AllTrails app, which can help a lot for this challenge. Simply download the app and it will help you to discover all the hikes and paths that surround your location (even when you are traveling!). It also ranks hikes based on difficulty, noting whether the route is easy, medium, or hard. This will help you to find a hike that matches your current skill level.**

→ **Start small with an easy hike then set a goal to tackle one of the more challenging hikes by the end of the 30 days!**

→ **Please practice safe hiking and always let a loved one know where you are going and when you expect to return. It's also a good idea to always hike with a friend and bring plenty of water.**

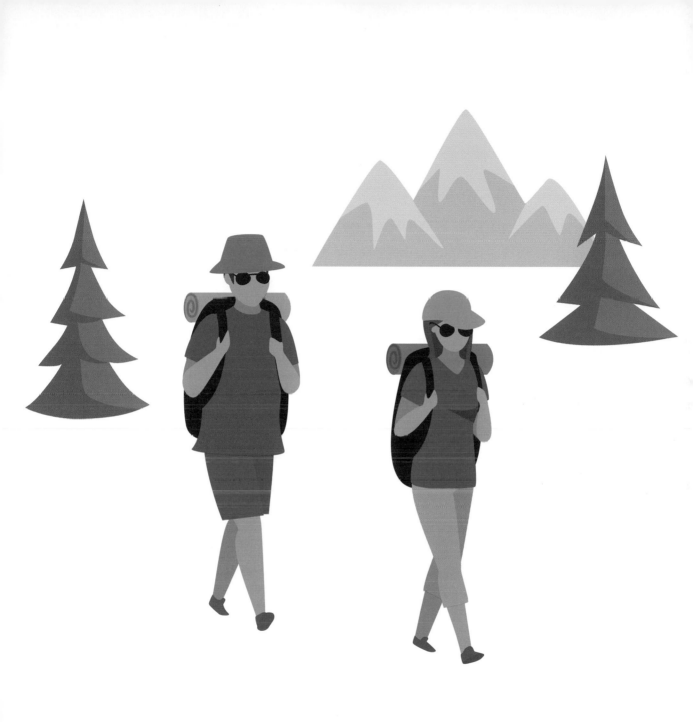

15. BE ACTIVE OUTDOORS

Our bodies and minds crave being outdoors. As you head outside and really take in the beauty that surrounds you, it is nearly impossible not to feel the energy shift within you. So why not use this natural desire to be outside to your advantage and get out and move!

This challenge will work best when the weather obliges. But even if you stumble upon a rainy day during your 30-day challenge, embrace it and use that day to dance in the rain! Whether you have 5 minutes or 60, the idea is to get outside every day and move for 30 days.

Here are some fun ways to tackle this challenge:

- → Bike ride
- → Rollerblade
- → Skateboard
- → Unicycle
- → Scooter
- → Meditate
- → Yoga
- → Walk
- → Run
- → Hike
- → Climb a tree
- → Disc golf
- → Throw a Frisbee with a friend
- → Tennis
- → Golf
- → Basketball
- → Four square
- → Head to the park and hit the swings!
- → Tetherball
- → Cricket
- → Baseball
- → Badminton
- → Croquet
- → Horseshoes
- → Shuffleboard
- → Hopscotch
- → Play tag
- → Play catch
- → Jump rope
- → Work on your cartwheel
- → Roller skate
- → Swim
- → Water-ski
- → Ski
- → Snowboard
- → Volleyball
- → Surf
- → Take your dog for a walk
- → Skip stones at the lake
- → Weed your yard
- → Mow your lawn

Once you're outside enjoying this beautiful planet we live on, you'll feel the benefits of an enhanced mood and a chance to smile, play, and laugh!

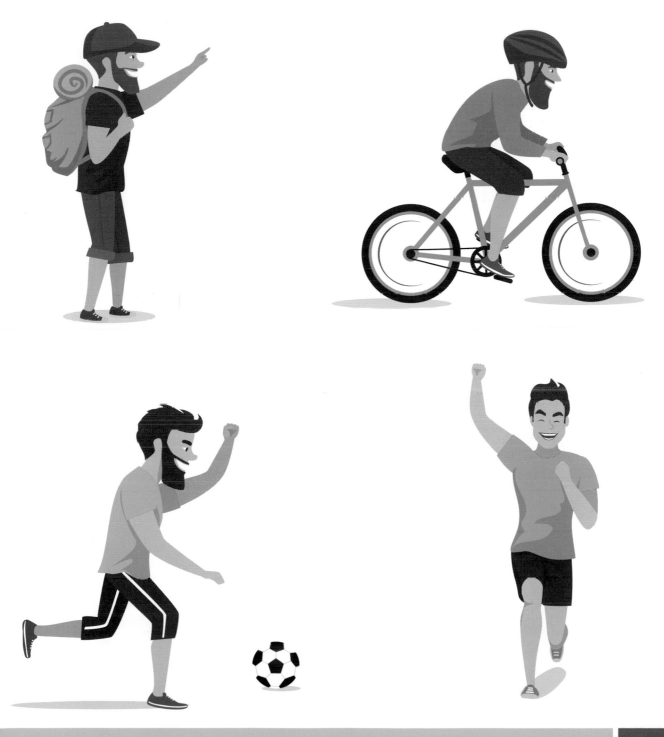

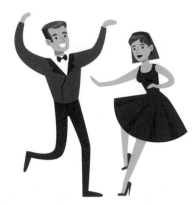
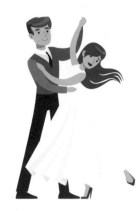
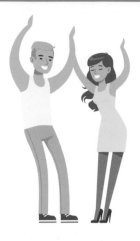
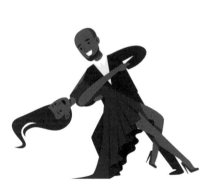
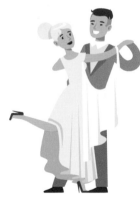
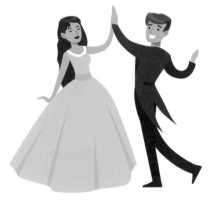
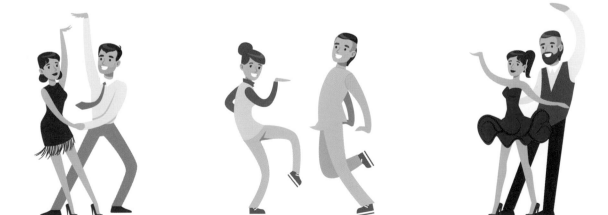

My kids love to dance. As soon as a song they like comes on, they can't help but start to move. They wiggle their bodies and move to the beat of the music with reckless abandon. It is so inspiring because they literally dance like no one is watching and you can feel their joy. Whether they are in time or on the beat doesn't matter at all. They dance for the fun of it. Kids are pretty cool that way.

This is my intention for you during this 30-day dance challenge. Let go of the need for perfection or "technique," and just feel the music and how it makes you move. Let the joy of music and dancing free you!

Here are some fun ways to incorporate dance into your daily routine for 30 days:

→ **Find a YouTube dance class**

→ **Crank your favorite jam and just go for it!**

→ **Go line-dancing with friends**

→ **Take a dance class**

PICK A NEW GENRE OF MUSIC EACH WEEK AND PERFECT YOUR MOVES. SOME IDEAS:

» '80s

» Country

» Hip-hop

» Boy bands

» '90s alternative

» Club mix

» Go out to a dance club (this is actually how I met my husband!)

Have fun with this challenge. Whether you let loose and dance for 5 minutes or dance the night away at a club, enjoy it! You might be surprised how much you miss it and your inner child is going to love you for it.

This SUPER challenge is not meant to overwhelm or scare you. I remember back when I first started working out and making my health a priority, I decided I would take it day by day. As that got easier, I transitioned to focusing on month by month.

Now all these years later, working out is just part of who I am. It sounds crazy, right? I would have laughed at me too. But I promise you that every day you choose to wake up and move you are getting closer to making exercising a part of who you are, and it's a habit that is pretty unshakable.

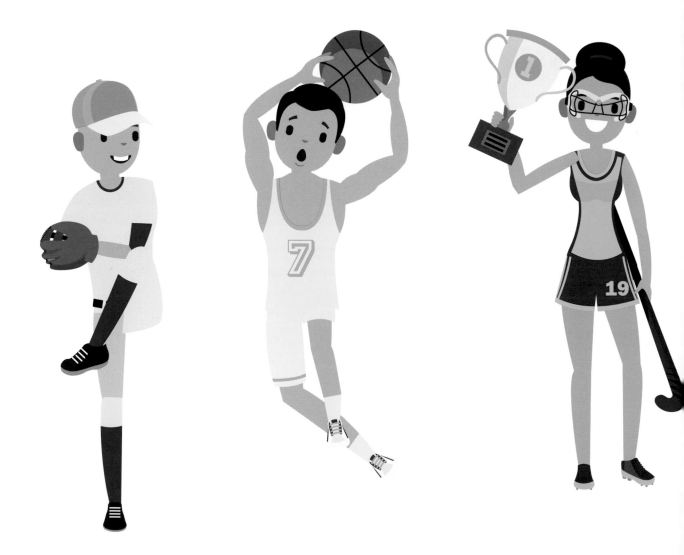

So every day for an entire year I will give you exercises to complete. As a beginner you can complete the exercises once and check "work out" off your to-do list for the day. As you become more used to the routine, you can move through the exercises three or four times. You'll be amazed by the improvement you see and feel. Stick with me for this amazing SUPER challenge. I will guide you through an entire year of making moving EVERY DAY a part of who you are! Let me know how you are doing by tagging me on social media using #andiemademedoit.

While the workout plans indicate the last two days of the week for play and rest, adjust your workouts as needed so those days fall on weekends if it is most convenient for your schedule. You'll need light dumbbells and a jump rope to complete many of the exercises. For exercises performed on both the right and left side of the body, like lunges, do the number of reps indicated on both sides before continuing. If you don't know how to do an exercise, go to www.maybeiwill.com/challengesbook for instructions.

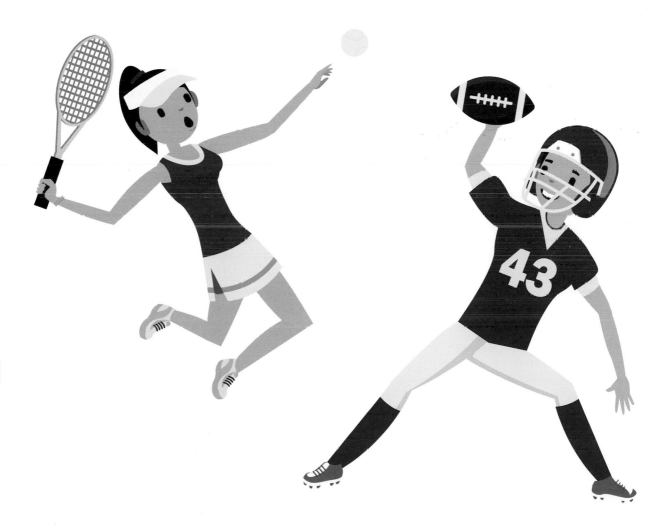

18. JUMP INTO JANUARY

The holidays are over. Maybe you've had a bit more eggnog/candy/fruitcake/cookies than you should have. Whether or not you make a New Year's resolution, you can start your year off right with this January challenge.

Note: While the workout plans here indicate the last two days of the week for play and rest, respectively, adjust your workouts as needed so those days fall on weekends if it is most convenient for your schedule. You'll need light dumbbells and a jump rope to complete many of the exercises. For exercises performed on both the right and left side of the body, like lunges, do the number of reps indicated on both sides before continuing. If you don't know how to do an exercise, go to www.maybeiwill.com/challengesbook for instructions.

Day 1: Chest and Triceps
1. **Push-Ups (5 to 10 reps)**
2. **Triceps Kickbacks (10 to 12 reps)**
3. **Chest Flies (10 to 12 reps)**
4. **Triceps Dips (10 to 12 reps)**

Day 2: Cardio
1. **Inch Worms (5 to 10 reps)**
2. **Froggers (5 to 10 reps)**
3. **Jumping Jacks (20 reps)**
4. **Ladders (20 seconds)**

Day 3: Back and Biceps
1. **Biceps Curls (10 to 12 reps)**
2. **Renegade Rows (10 to 12 reps)**
3. **Hammer Curls (10 to 12 reps)**
4. **Bent-Over Flies (10 to 12 reps)**

Day 4: Cardio
Go for a walk (20 to 30 minutes)

Day 5: Legs
1. **Sumo Squats (10 to 12 reps)**
2. **Curtsy Lunges (10 to 12 reps)**
3. **Donkey Kicks (10 to 12 reps)**
4. **Side Leg Lifts (10 to 12 reps)**

Day 6: Be Active
Saturdays are for playing and being active.

Day 7: Rest
Sundays are your rest days!

Day 8: Abs and Shoulders
1. **Sit-Ups (10 to 20 reps)**
2. **Milk Pours (10 to 12 reps)**
3. **Plank (30 to 60 seconds)**
4. **Overhead Presses (10 to 12 reps)**

Day 9: Cardio
1. **Skaters (30 to 60 seconds)**
2. **Jumping Lunges (10 to 12 reps)**
3. **Four Corners (30 to 60 seconds)**
4. **Jump Squats (10 to 12 reps)**

Day 10: Chest and Triceps
1. **Diamond Push-Ups (5 to 10 reps)**
2. **Chest Presses (10 to 12 reps)**
3. **Skull Crushers (10 to 12 reps)**
4. **Push-Ups (5 to 10 reps)**

Day 11: Cardio
Go for a walk (25 to 30 minutes)

Day 12: Back and Biceps
1. **7s (3 sets)**
2. **Supermans (10 to 12 reps)**
3. **W Curls (10 to 12 reps)**
4. **Seated Rows (10 to 12 reps)**

Day 13: Be Active
Depending on where you live, this may be a good day to go skiing!

Day 14: Rest

Day 15: Legs
1. **Fire Hydrants (10 to 12 reps)**
2. **Squats (10 to 12 reps)**
3. **Side Lunges (10 to 12 reps)**
4. **Deadlifts (10 to 12 reps)**

Day 16: Cardio
1. **Jump Rope (30 to 60 seconds)**
2. **Windmills (10 to 12 reps)**
3. **Jump Rope (30 to 60 seconds)**
4. **Kickboxing Kicks (10 to 12 reps)**

Day 17: Abs and Shoulders

1. V-Ups (10 to 12 reps)
2. Upright Rows (10 to 12 reps)
3. Mason Twists (10 to 12 reps)
4. T Raises (10 to 12 reps)

Day 18: Cardio

Go for a walk (25 to 30 minutes). Try adding in a burst of jogging.

Day 19: Chest and Triceps

1. Overhead Triceps Extensions (10 to 12 reps)
2. Incline Push-Ups (10 to 12 reps)
3. Triceps Kickbacks (10 to 12 reps)
4. Alternating Chest Flies (10 to 12 reps)

Day 20: Be Active

Depending on where you live, maybe try snowshoeing or sledding.

Day 21: Rest

Day 22: Back and Biceps

1. Biceps Curls (10 to 12 reps)
2. Bent-Over Rows (10 to 12 reps)
3. Concentration Curls (10 to 12 reps)
4. Bent-Over Flies (10 to 12 reps)

Day 23: Cardio

1. Burpees (5 to 10 reps)
2. Crab Walks (30 to 60 seconds)
3. Jumping Jacks (10 to 12 reps)
4. Bear Walks (30 to 60 seconds)

Day 24: Legs

1. Sumo Squats (10 to 12 reps)
2. Reverse Lunges (10 to 12 reps)
3. Bridges (10 to 12 reps, each with a 20-second hold at the top of the movement)
4. Leg Lifts (10 to 12 reps)

Day 25: Cardio (Repeat 2 or 3 times)

1. Jump Rope (30 to 60 seconds); rest 20 seconds
2. Jump Rope (30 to 60 seconds); rest 20 seconds

Day 26: Abs and Shoulders

1. Roll-Ups (10 reps)
2. Milk Pours (10 to 12 reps)
3. Starfishes (10 reps)
4. Overhead Presses (10 to 12 reps)

Day 27: Be Active

Depending on where you live, maybe go snowshoeing today.

Day 28: Rest

Day 29: Chest and Triceps

1. Push-Ups (10 to 12 reps)
2. Skull Crushers (10 to 12 reps)
3. Chest Flies (10 to 12 reps)
4. Triceps Dips (10 to 12 reps)

Day 30: Cardio

1. Mummy Kicks (30 to 60 seconds)
2. Squat Thrusts (10 to 12 reps)
3. Four Corners (30 to 60 seconds)
4. High Knees (10 to 12 reps)

Day 31: Back and Biceps

1. W Curls (10 to 12 reps)
2. Renegade Rows (10 to 12 reps)
3. 7s (3 sets)
4. Seated Rows (10 to 12 reps)

19. FAST FORWARD INTO FEBRUARY

Happy Valentine's Day! Fall in love with fitness and taking care of *you* this month.

Note: While the workout plans here indicate the last two days of the week for play and rest, respectively, adjust your workouts as needed so those days fall on weekends if it is most convenient for your schedule. You'll need light dumbbells and a jump rope to complete many of the exercises. For exercises performed on both the right and left side of the body, like lunges, do the number of reps indicated on both sides before continuing. If you don't know how to do an exercise, go to www.maybeiwill.com/challengesbook for instructions.

Day 1: Legs
1. Donkey Kicks (10 to 12 reps)
2. Fire Hydrants (10 to 12 reps)
3. Deadlifts (10 to 12 reps)
4. Squats (10 to 12 reps)

Day 2: Cardio (Repeat 2 or 3 times)
1. Jumping Jacks (20 reps)
2. Inch Worms (5 to 10 reps)
3. Jumping Jacks (20 reps)
4. Inch Worms (5 to 10 reps)

Day 3: Abs and Shoulders
1. Crunches (15 to 30 reps)
2. Upright Rows (10 to 12 reps)
3. Side Bends (20 reps)
4. Arm Circles (10 to 12 reps)

Day 4: Cardio (Repeat 2 or 3 times)
1. Ladders (30 to 60 seconds); rest 20 seconds
2. Mountain Climbers (30 to 60 seconds); rest 20 seconds

Day 5: Chest and Triceps
1. Triceps Kickbacks (10 to 12 reps)
2. Incline Push-Ups (10 to 12 reps)
3. Diamond Push-Ups (10 to 12 reps)
4. Chest Presses (10 to 12 reps)

Day 6: Be Active
Depending on where you live, maybe go ice-skating today.

Day 7: Rest

Day 8: Back and Biceps
1. Supermans (10 to 12 reps)
2. Biceps Curls (10 to 12 reps)
3. Bent-Over Flies (10 to 12 reps)
4. W Curls (10 to 12 reps)

Day 9: Cardio
1. Burpees (5 to 10 reps)
2. Inch Worms (5 to 10 reps)
3. Jumping Lunges (10 to 12 reps)
4. Windmills (10 to 20 reps)

Day 10: Legs
1. Side Lunges (10 to 12 reps)
2. Side Leg Lifts (10 to 12 reps)
3. Curtsy Squats (10 to 12 reps)
4. Plie Squats (10 to 12 reps)

Day 11: Cardio (Repeat 2 or 3 times)
1. Crab Walks (30 to 60 seconds)
2. Kickboxing Kicks (20 reps)
3. Bear Walks (30 to 60 seconds)
4. Rear Kicks (20 reps)

Day 12: Abs and Shoulders
1. V-Ups (10 to 12 reps)
2. T Raises (10 to 12 reps)
3. Criss Cross (20 reps)
4. Milk Pours (10 to 12 reps)

Day 13: Be Active
Go for a brisk walk outside.

Day 14: Rest

Day 15: Chest and Triceps

1. Triceps Dips (10 to 12 reps)
2. Chest Flies (10 to 12 reps)
3. Overhead Triceps Extensions (10 to 12 reps)
4. Chest Presses (10 to 12 reps)

Day 16: Cardio (Repeat 2 or 3 times)

1. Jump Rope (30 to 60 seconds); rest 20 seconds
2. Jump Rope (30 to 60 seconds); rest 20 seconds

Day 17: Back and Biceps

1. Bent-Over Rows (10 to 12 reps)
2. 7s (repeat 3 times)
3. Supermans (10 to 12 reps)
4. Concentration Curls (10 to 12 reps)

Day 18: Cardio

1. Four Corners (30 to 60 seconds)
2. Jump Squats (10 to 12 reps)
3. Mountain Climbers (30 to 60 seconds)
4. Jumping Lunges (10 to 12 reps)

Day 19: Legs

1. Deadlifts (10 to 12 reps)
2. Bridges (10 to 12 reps, each with a 20-second hold at the top of the movement)
3. Plie Squats (10 to 12 reps)
4. Calf Raises (10 to 12 reps, each with a 20-second hold at the top of the movement)

Day 20: Be Active

Try playing Frisbee or tennis.

Day 21: Rest

Day 22: Abs and Shoulders

1. Shoulder Shrugs (10 to 15 reps)
2. Heel Touches (20 reps)
3. Upright Rows (10 to 12 reps)
4. Plank (30 to 60 seconds)

Day 23: Cardio (Repeat 2 or 3 times)

1. Skaters (30 to 60 seconds)
2. Windmills (10 to 20 reps)
3. Skaters (30 to 60 seconds)
4. Inch Worms (10 to 15 reps)

Day 24: Chest and Triceps

1. Push-Ups (10 to 12 reps)
2. Triceps Kickbacks (10 to 12 reps)
3. Chest Flies (10 to 12 reps)
4. Skull Crushers (10 to 12 reps)

Day 25: Cardio (Repeat 2 or 3 times)

1. Heismans (30 to 60 seconds); rest 10 seconds
2. Ladders (30 to 60 seconds); rest 10 seconds

Day 26: Back and Biceps

1. Biceps Curls (10 to 12 reps)
2. Seated Rows (10 to 12 reps)
3. Hammer Curls (10 to 12 reps)
4. Renegade Rows (10 to 12 reps)

Day 27: Be Active

Go for a bike ride.

Day 28: Rest

20. MOVE IT MARCH

Keep your goal roaring like a lion throughout March. The spring equinox toward the latter end of the month signifies a shift to longer days and more daylight hours for movement and exercise.

Note: While the workout plans here indicate the last two days of the week for play and rest, respectively, adjust your workouts as needed so those days fall on weekends if it is most convenient for your schedule. You'll need light dumbbells and a jump rope to complete many of the exercises. For exercises performed on both the right and left side of the body, like lunges, do the number of reps indicated on both sides before continuing. If you don't know how to do an exercise, go to www.maybeiwill.com/challengesbook for instructions.

Day 1: Legs
1. **Fire Hydrants (10 to 12 reps)**
2. **Sumo Squats (10 to 12 reps)**
3. **Donkey Kicks (10 to 12 reps)**
4. **Curtsy Squats (10 to 12 reps)**

Day 2: Cardio (Repeat 2 or 3 times)
1. **Mountain Climbers (30 to 60 seconds)**
2. **Inch Worms (5 to 10 reps)**
3. **High Knees (10 to 12 reps)**
4. **Kickboxing Kicks (30 to 60 seconds)**

Day 3: Abs and Shoulders
1. **Swimmers (100 counts)**
2. **V Raises (10 to 12 reps)**
3. **Roll-Ups (10 to 12 reps)**
4. **Pike Push-Ups (10 to 12 reps)**

Day 4: Cardio (Repeat 2 or 3 times)
1. **Heismans (30 to 60 seconds)**
2. **Jumping Lunges (10 to 12 reps)**
3. **Froggers (30 to 60 seconds)**
4. **Squats Thrusts (10 to 12 reps)**

Day 5: Chest and Triceps
1. **Push-Ups (10 to 12 reps)**
2. **Triceps Dips (10 to 12 reps)**
3. **Chest Flies (10 to 12 reps)**
4. **Overhead Triceps Extensions (10 to 12 reps)**

Day 6: Be Active
Fly a kite.

Day 7: Rest

Day 8: Back and Biceps
1. **Upper Curls (10 to 12 reps)**
2. **Supermans (10 to 12 reps)**
3. **Lower Curls (10 to 12 reps)**
4. **Bent-Over Rows (10 to 12 reps)**

Day 9: Cardio (Repeat 2 or 3 times)
1. **Jumping Jacks (20 reps)**
2. **Inch Worms (5 to 10 reps)**
3. **Jumping Jacks (20 reps)**
4. **Inch Worms (5 to 10 reps)**

Day 10: Legs
1. **Reverse Lunges (10 to 12 reps)**
2. **Step-Ups (10 to 12 reps)**
3. **Deadlifts (10 to 12 reps)**
4. **Bridges (10 to 12 reps, each with a 20-second hold at the top of the movement)**

Day 11: Cardio (Repeat 2 or 3 times)
1. **Skaters (20 reps); rest 10 seconds**
2. **Burpees (10 to 12 reps); rest 10 seconds**

Day 12: Abs and Shoulders
1. **Mason Twists (10 to 12 reps)**
2. **Milk Pours (10 to 12 reps)**
3. **V-Ups (10 to 12 reps)**
4. **Upright Rows (10 to 12 reps)**

Day 13: Be Active
Go for a hike.

Day 14: Rest

Day 15: Chest and Triceps

1. **Incline Push-Ups (10 to 12 reps)**
2. **Skull Crushers (10 to 12 reps)**
3. **Chest Presses (10 to 12 reps)**
4. **Triceps Kickbacks (10 to 12 reps)**

Day 16: Cardio (Repeat 2 or 3 times)

1. **Jump Rope (30 to 60 seconds); rest 10 seconds**
2. **Jump Rope (30 to 60 seconds); rest 10 seconds**

Day 17: Back and Biceps

1. **7s (3 sets)**
2. **Renegade Rows (10 to 12 reps)**
3. **Hammer Curls (10 to 12 reps)**
4. **Seated Rows (10 to 15 reps)**

Day 18: Cardio (Repeat 2 or 3 times)

1. **High Knees (10 to 12 reps)**
2. **Ladders (20 to 30 seconds)**
3. **Froggers (10 to 12 reps)**
4. **Mountain Climbers (20 to 30 seconds)**

Day 19: Legs

1. **Squats (10 to 12 reps)**
2. **Surrenders (10 to 12 reps)**
3. **Curtsy Squats (10 to 12 reps)**
4. **Side Lunges (10 to 12 reps)**

Day 20: Be Active

Explore your city on foot.

Day 21: Rest Day

Day 22: Abs and Shoulders

1. **Plank (30 to 60 seconds)**
2. **Shoulder Shrugs (10 to 12 reps)**
3. **Bird Dogs (10 to 12 reps)**
4. **Overhead Presses (10 to 12 reps)**

Day 23: Cardio (Repeat 2 or 3 times)

1. **Burpees (10 to 12 reps)**
2. **Inch Worms (10 to 12 reps)**
3. **Burpees (10 to 12 reps)**
4. **Windmills (10 to 12 reps)**

Day 24: Chest and Triceps

1. **Chest Presses (10 to 12 reps)**
2. **Triceps Dips (10 to 12 reps)**
3. **Chest Flies (10 to 12 reps)**
4. **Diamond Push-Ups (10 to 15 reps)**

Day 25: Cardio (Repeat 2 or 3 times)

1. **Heismans (30 to 60 seconds); rest 10 seconds**
2. **Jumping Jacks (30 to 60 seconds); rest 10 seconds**

Day 26: Back and Biceps

1. **W Curls (10 or 12 reps)**
2. **Supermans (10 or 12 reps)**
3. **Biceps Curls (10 or 12 reps)**
4. **Bent-Over Flies (10 or 12 reps)**

Day 27: Be Active

Play a round of mini golf.

Day 28: Rest

Day 29: Leg Day

1. **Walking Lunges (10 to 12 reps)**
2. **Side Lunges (10 to 12 reps)**
3. **Bridges (10 to 12 reps, each with a 20-second hold at the top of the movement)**
4. **Plie Squats (10 to 12 reps)**

Day 30: Cardio (Repeat 2 or 3 times)

1. **Froggers (30 to 60 seconds)**
2. **Inch Worms (10 to 12 reps)**
3. **Four Corners (30 to 60 seconds)**
4. **Jumping Lunges (10 to 12 reps)**

Day 31: Abs and Shoulders

1. **Starfishes (10 to 12 reps)**
2. **T Raises (10 to 12 reps)**
3. **Trunk Rotations (20 reps)**
4. **Weighted Arm Circles (10 to 12 reps)**

21. ACCELERATE INTO APRIL

Don't let April showers rain all over your goals! Most of the exercises below can be done indoors.

Note: While the workout plans here indicate the last two days of the week for play and rest, respectively, adjust your workouts as needed so those days fall on weekends if it is most convenient for your schedule. You'll need light dumbbells and a jump rope to complete many of the exercises. For exercises performed on both the right and left side of the body, like lunges, do the number of reps indicated on both sides before continuing. If you don't know how to do an exercise, go to www.maybeiwill.com/challengesbook for instructions.

Day 1: Chest and Triceps
1. **Push-Ups (10 to 12 reps)**
2. **Skull Crushers (10 to 12 reps)**
3. **Chest Presses (10 to 12 reps)**
4. **Diamond Push-Ups (10 to 12 reps)**

Day 2: Cardio (Repeat 2 or 3 times)
1. **Jumping Rope (30 to 60 seconds); rest 10 seconds**
2. **Jumping Rope (30 to 60 seconds); rest 10 seconds**

Day 3: Back and Biceps
1. **7s (3 sets)**
2. **Bent-Over Rows (10 to 12 reps)**
3. **Hammer Curls (10 to 12 reps)**
4. **Supermans (10 to 12 reps)**

Day 4: Cardio (Repeat 2 or 3 times)
1. **Skaters (10 to 12 reps)**
2. **Jumping Lunges (10 to 12 reps)**
3. **Inch Worms (10 to 12 reps)**
4. **Skaters (10 to 12 reps)**

Day 5: Legs
1. **Step-Ups (10 to 12 reps)**
2. **Deadlifts (10 to 12 reps)**
3. **Lunges (10 to 12 reps)**
4. **Sumo Squats (10 to 12 reps)**

Day 6: Be Active
Grab a basketball and play PIG or HORSE.

Day 7: Rest Day

Day 8: Abs and Shoulders
1. **Swimmers (100 counts)**
2. **Overhead Presses (10 to 12 reps)**
3. **Roll-Ups (10 to 12 reps)**
4. **Milk Pours (10 to 12 reps)**

Day 9: Cardio (Repeat 2 or 3 times)
1. **Froggers (10 to 12 reps)**
2. **Four Squares (30 to 60 seconds)**
3. **Jump Squats (10 to 12 reps)**
4. **Froggers (10 to 12 reps)**

Day 10: Chest and Triceps
1. **Chest Flies (10 to 12 reps)**
2. **Triceps Dips (10 to 12 reps)**
3. **Incline Push-Ups (10 to 12 reps)**
4. **Overhead Triceps Extensions (10 to 12 reps)**

Day 11: Cardio (Repeat 2 or 3 times)
1. **Burpees (30 to 60 seconds); rest 10 seconds**
2. **Burpees (30 to 60 seconds); rest 10 seconds**

Day 12: Back and Biceps
1. **W Biceps Curls (10 to 12 reps)**
2. **Seated Rows (10 to 12 reps)**
3. **Biceps Curls (10 to 12 reps)**
4. **Lat Pulls (10 to 12 reps)**

Day 13: Be Active
Try a dance class.

Day 14: Rest

Day 15: Leg
1. **Donkey Kicks (10 to 12 reps)**
2. **Fire Hydrants (10 to 12 reps)**
3. **Deadlifts (10 to 12 reps)**
4. **Side Lunges (10 to 12 reps)**

Day 16: Cardio (Repeat 2 or 3 times)

1. Inch Worms (10 to 12 reps)
2. Windmills (10 to 12 reps)
3. Surrenders (10 to 12 reps)
4. Jumping Jacks (30 to 60 seconds)

Day 17: Abs and Shoulders

1. Crunches (20 to 30 reps)
2. Shoulder Shrugs (10 to 12 reps)
3. Criss Crosses (10 to 12 reps)
4. Weighted Arm Circles (10 to 12 reps)

Day 18: Cardio (Repeat 2 or 3 times)

1. Jumping Rope (30 to 60 seconds); rest 10 seconds
2. Jumping Rope (30 to 60 seconds); rest 10 seconds

Day 19: Chest and Triceps

1. Chest Presses (10 to 12 reps)
2. Triceps Kickbacks (10 to 12 reps)
3. Push-Ups (10 to 12 reps)
4. Diamond Push-Ups (10 to 12 reps)

Day 20: Be Active

Pack a picnic and head outside.

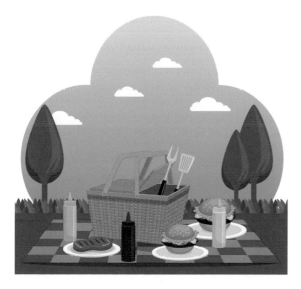

Day 21: Rest Day

Day 22: Back and Biceps

1. Hammer Curls (10 to 12 reps)
2. Supermans (10 to 12 reps)
3. Concentration Curls (10 to 12 reps)
4. Bent-Over Flies (10 to 12 reps)

Day 23: Cardio (Repeat 2 or 3 times)

1. Jumping Jacks (20 to 30 seconds)
2. Burpees (10 to 12 reps)
3. Mountain Climbers (10 to 12 reps)
4. Windmills (10 to 12 reps)

Day 24: Legs

1. Reverse Lunges (10 to 12 reps)
2. Sumo Squats (10 to 12 reps)
3. Step-Ups (10 to 12 reps)
4. Curtsy Squats (10 to 12 reps)

Day 25: Cardio (Repeat 2 or 3 times)

1. Four Squares (30 to 60 seconds)
2. Inch Worms (10 to 12 reps)
3. Four Squares (30 to 60 seconds)
4. Inch Worms (10 to 12 reps)

Day 26: Abs and Shoulders

1. V-Ups (10 to 12 reps)
2. Upright Rows (10 to 12 reps)
3. Starfishes (10 to 12 reps)
4. V Raises (10 to 12 reps)

Day 27: Be Active

Go roller blading!

Day 28: Rest Day

Day 29: Chest and Triceps

1. Incline Push-Ups (10 to 12 reps)
2. Skull Crushers (10 to 12 reps)
3. Chest Flies (10 to 12 reps)
4. Triceps Dips (10 to 12 reps)

Day 30: Cardio (Repeat 2 or 3 times)

1. Kickboxing Kicks (20 to 30 seconds)
2. Squat Thrusts (10 to 12 reps)
3. Ladders (10 to 12 reps)
4. Crab Walks (20 to 30 seconds)

22. MOTIVATED MAY

Summer is almost here—stay focused and keep going, you, rock star, you!

Note: While the workout plans here indicate the last two days of the week for play and rest, respectively, adjust your workouts as needed so those days fall on weekends if it is most convenient for your schedule. You'll need light dumbbells and a jump rope to complete many of the exercises. For exercises performed on both the right and left side of the body, like lunges, do the number of reps indicated on both sides before continuing. If you don't know how to do an exercise, go to www.maybeiwill.com/challengesbook for instructions.

Day 1: Back and Biceps
1. 7s (3 sets)
2. Lat Pulls (10 to 12 reps)
3. Hammer Curls (10 to 12 reps)
4. Seated Rows (10 to 12 reps)

Day 2: Cardio (Repeat 2 or 3 times)
1. Jump Rope (30 to 60 seconds); rest 10 seconds
2. Jump Rope (30 to 60 seconds); rest 10 seconds

Day 3: Legs
1. Squats (10 to 12 reps)
2. Lunges (10 to 12 reps)
3. Plie Squats (10 to 12 reps)
4. Side Lunges (10 to 12 reps)

Day 4: Cardio (Repeat 2 or 3 times)
1. Skaters (10 to 12 reps)
2. Jumping Lunges (10 to 12 reps)
3. Four Squares (10 to 12 reps)
4. Jump Squats (10 to 12 reps)

Day 5: Abs and Shoulders
1. Plank (30 to 60 seconds)
2. T Raises (10 to 12 reps)
3. Swimmers (100 counts)
4. Milk Pours (10 to 12 reps)

Day 6: Be Active

Try a yoga class.

Day 7: Rest Day

Day 8: Chest and Triceps
1. Push-Ups (10 to 12 reps)
2. Triceps Dips (10 to 12 reps)
3. Chest Presses (10 to 12 reps)
4. Skull Crushers (10 to 12 reps)

Day 9: Cardio (Repeat 2 or 3 times)
1. Mountain Climbers (30 to 60 seconds); rest 10 seconds
2. Mountain Climbers (30 to 60 seconds); rest 10 seconds

Day 10: Back and Biceps
1. L Curls (10 to 12 reps)
2. Supermans (10 to 12 reps)
3. W Curls (10 to 12 reps)
4. Bent-Over Rows (10 to 12 reps)

Day 11: Cardio (Repeat 2 or 3 times)
1. Ladders (10 to 12 reps)
2. Jumping Jacks (15 to 20 reps)
3. Mountain Climbers (10 to 12 reps)
4. Kickboxing Kicks (15 to 20 reps)

Day 12: Legs
1. Leg Lifts (10 to 12 reps)
2. Donkey Kicks (10 to 12 reps)
3. Fire Hydrants (10 to 12 reps)
4. Curtsy Squats (10 to 12 reps)

Day 13: Be Active

Go out dancing!

Day 14: Rest Day

Day 15: Abs and Shoulders

1. **Plank (30 to 60 seconds)**
2. **V Raises (10 to 12 reps)**
3. **Starfishes (10 to 12 reps)**
4. **Upright Row (10 to 12 reps)**

Day 16: Cardio (Repeat 2 or 3 times)

1. **Skaters (10 to 12 reps)**
2. **Surrenders (10 to 12 reps)**
3. **Inch Worms (10 to 12 reps)**
4. **Skaters (10 to 12 reps)**

Day 17: Chest and Triceps

1. **Chest Flies (10 to 12 reps)**
2. **Triceps Dips (10 to 12 reps)**
3. **Chest Presses (10 to 12 reps)**
4. **Triceps Kickbacks (10 to 12 reps)**

Day 18: Cardio (Repeat 2 or 3 times)

1. **Jump Rope (30 to 60 seconds); rest 10 seconds**
2. **Jump Rope (30 to 60 seconds); rest 10 seconds**

Day 19: Back and Biceps

1. **7s (3 sets)**
2. **Seated Rows (10 to 12 reps)**
3. **Biceps Curls (10 to 12 reps)**
4. **Lat Pulls (10 to 12 reps)**

Day 20: Be Active

Go bowling.

Day 21: Rest Day

Day 22: Legs

1. **Step-Ups (10 to 12 reps)**
2. **Deadlifts (10 to 12 reps)**
3. **Side Lunges (10 to 12 reps)**
4. **Sumo Squats (10 to 12 reps)**

Day 23: Cardio (Repeat 2 or 3 times)

1. **Mountain Climbers (10 to 12 reps)**
2. **Ladders (10 to 12 reps)**
3. **Froggers (10 to 12 reps)**
4. **Burpees (10 to 12 reps)**

Day 24: Abs and Shoulders

1. **V-Ups (10 to 12 reps)**
2. **Overhead Shoulder Presses (10 to 12 reps)**
3. **Criss Crosses (15 to 20 reps)**
4. **T Raises (10 to 12 reps)**

Day 25: Cardio (Repeat 2 or 3 times)

1. **Jumping Jacks (20 to 30 reps)**
2. **Inch Worms (10 to 12 reps)**
3. **Froggers (10 to 12 reps)**
4. **Inch Worms (10 to 12 reps)**

Day 26: Chest and Triceps

1. **Incline Push-Ups (10 to 12 reps)**
2. **Overhead Triceps Extensions (10 to 12 reps)**
3. **Chest Flies (10 to 12 reps)**
4. **Diamond Push-Ups (10 to 12 reps)**

Day 27: Be Active

Try water-skiing.

Day 28: Rest Day

Day 29: Back and Biceps

1. **Biceps Curls (10 to 12 reps)**
2. **Bent-Over Flies (10 to 12 reps)**
3. **Concentration Curls (10 to 12 reps)**
4. **Supermans (10 to 12 reps)**

Day 30: Cardio (Repeat 2 or 3 times)

1. **Jump Rope (30 to 60 seconds); rest 10 seconds**
2. **Jump Rope (30 to 60 seconds); rest 10 seconds**

Day 31: Legs

1. **Step-Ups (10 to 12 reps)**
2. **Deadlifts (10 to 12 reps)**
3. **Side Lunges (10 to 12 reps)**
4. **Curtsy Lunges (10 to 12 reps)**

23. JOYOUS JUNE

Summer's here—take your workout into your backyard or a local park.

Note: While the workout plans here indicate the last two days of the week for play and rest, respectively, adjust your workouts as needed so those days fall on weekends if it is most convenient for your schedule. You'll need light dumbbells and a jump rope to complete many of the exercises. For exercises performed on both the right and left side of the body, like lunges, do the number of reps indicated on both sides before continuing. If you don't know how to do an exercise, go to www.maybeiwill.com/challengesbook for instructions.

Day 1: Abs and Shoulders
1. **Mason Twists (10 to 12 reps)**
2. **Shoulder Shrugs (10 to 12 reps)**
3. **Plank (30 to 60 seconds)**
4. **Milk Pours (10 to 12 reps)**

Day 2: Cardio (Repeat 2 or 3 times)
1. **Kickboxing Kicks (20 to 30 reps)**
2. **Surrenders (10 to 12 reps)**
3. **Inch Worms (10 to 12 reps)**
4. **Kickboxing Kicks (20 to 30 reps)**

Day 3: Chest and Triceps
1. **Chest Flies (10 to 15 reps)**
2. **Diamond Push-Ups (10 to 15 reps)**
3. **Chest Presses (10 to 15 reps)**
4. **Triceps Dips (10 to 15 reps)**

Day 4: Cardio (Repeat 2 or 3 times)
1. **Burpees (45 to 90 seconds); rest 10 seconds**
2. **Burpees (45 to 90 seconds); rest 10 seconds**

Day 5: Back and Biceps
1. **Concentration Curls (10 to 15 reps)**
2. **Supermans (10 to 15 reps)**
3. **Hammer Curls (10 to 15 reps)**
4. **Seated Rows (10 to 15 reps)**

Day 6: Be Active

Go geocaching.

Day 7: Rest Day

Day 8: Legs
1. **Donkey Kicks (10 to 15 reps)**
2. **Fire Hydrants (10 to 15 reps)**
3. **Side Lunges (10 to 15 reps)**
4. **Curtsy Squats (10 to 15 reps)**

Day 9: Cardio (Repeat 2 or 3 times)
1. **Surrenders (10 to 15 reps)**
2. **Inch Worms (10 to 15 reps)**
3. **Jumping Jacks (30 reps)**
4. **Jumping Lunges (10 to 15 reps)**

Day 10: Abs and Shoulders
1. **Swimmers (100 counts)**
2. **Milk Pours (10 to 15 reps)**
3. **Roll-Ups (10 to 15 reps)**
4. **T Raises (10 to 15 reps)**

Day 11: Cardio (Repeat 2 or 3 times)
1. **Mountain Climbers (45 to 90 seconds); rest 10 seconds**
2. **Mountain Climbers (45 to 90 seconds); rest 10 seconds**

Day 12: Chest to Triceps
1. **Incline Push-Ups (10 to 15 reps)**
2. **Triceps Kickbacks (10 to 15 reps)**
3. **Chest Presses (10 to 15 reps)**
4. **Triceps Dips (10 to 15 reps)**

Day 13: Be Active

Play a game of catch.

Day 14: Rest Day

Day 15: Back and Biceps
1. **W Curls (10 to 15 reps)**
2. **Lat Pulls (10 to 15 reps)**
3. **Hammer Curls (10 to 15 reps)**
4. **Bent-Over Flies (10 to 15 reps)**

Day 16: Cardio (Repeat 2 or 3 times)

1. **Jumping Jacks (20 to 30 reps)**
2. **High Knees (10 to 15 reps)**
3. **Windmills (20 to 30 reps)**
4. **Squat Thrusts (10 to 15 reps)**

Day 17: Legs

1. **Side Lunges (10 to 12 reps)**
2. **Plie Squats (10 to 12 reps)**
3. **Reverse Lunges (10 to 12 reps)**
4. **Sumo Squats (10 to 12 reps)**

Day 18: Cardio (Repeat 2 or 3 times)

1. **Froggers (10 to 15 reps)**
2. **Surrenders 10 to 15 reps)**
3. **Inch Worms (10 to 15 reps)**
4. **Ladders (10 to 15 reps)**

Day 19: Abs and Shoulders

1. **Crunches (20 to 30 reps)**
2. **Weighted Punches (10 to 15 reps)**
3. **Leg Raises (10 to 15 reps)**
4. **Milk Pours (10 to 15 reps)**

Day 20: Be Active

Try skateboarding or scootering.

Day 21: Rest Day

Day 22: Chest and Triceps

1. **Chest Presses (10 to 15 reps)**
2. **Triceps Overhead Extensions (10 to 15 reps)**
3. **Chest Flies (10 to 15 reps)**
4. **Skull Crushers (10 to 15 reps)**

Day 23: Cardio (Repeat 2 or 3 times)

1. **Skaters (10 to 15 reps)**
2. **Four Squares (10 to 15 reps)**
3. **Froggers (10 to 15 reps)**
4. **Jumping Lunges (10 to 15 reps)**

Day 24: Back and Biceps

1. **7s (3 sets)**
2. **Supermans (10 to 15 reps)**
3. **Hammer Curls (10 to 15 reps)**
4. **Renegade Rows (10 to 15 reps)**

Day 25: Cardio (Repeat 2 or 3 times)

1. **Heismans (45 to 90 seconds); rest 10 seconds**
2. **Heismans (45 to 90 seconds); rest 10 seconds**

Day 26: Legs

1. **Step-Ups (10 to 15 reps)**
2. **Bridges (10 to 15 reps, each with a 30-second hold at the top of the movement)**
3. **Deadlifts (10 to 15 reps)**
4. **Side Lunges (10 to 15 reps)**

Day 27: Be Active

Play hopscotch.

Day 28: Rest Day

Day 29: Abs and Shoulders

1. **Plank (45 to 90 seconds)**
2. **Shoulder Shrugs (10 to 15 reps)**
3. **Swimmers (100 counts)**
4. **V Raises (10 to 15 seconds)**

Day 30: Cardio (Repeat 2 or 3 times)

1. **Kickboxing Kicks (20 to 30 reps)**
2. **Jump Squats (10 to 15 reps)**
3. **Windmills (20 to 30 reps)**
4. **Jumping Lunges (10 to 15 reps)**

24. JAZZY JULY

You're a firework—get up and get moving! Even if you are on vacation, find a beach, park, or hotel gym to fit in your fitness fix. If you don't have access to weights, canned goods or water bottles can work in a pinch.

Note: While the workout plans here indicate the last two days of the week for play and rest, respectively, adjust your workouts as needed so those days fall on weekends if it is most convenient for your schedule. You'll need light dumbbells and a jump rope to complete many of the exercises. For exercises performed on both the right and left side of the body, like lunges, do the number of reps indicated on both sides before continuing. If you don't know how to do an exercise, go to www.maybeiwill.com/challengesbook for instructions.

Day 1: Chest and Triceps
1. **Push-Ups (10 to 15 reps)**
2. **Triceps Dips (10 to 15 reps)**
3. **Incline Push-Ups (10 to 15 reps)**
4. **Diamond Push-Ups (10 to 15 reps)**

Day 2: Cardio (Repeat 2 or 3 times)
1. **Windmills (20 to 30 reps)**
2. **Wide Arm Circles (20 to 30 reps)**
3. **Skaters (10 to 15 reps)**
4. **Windmills (20 to 30 reps)**

Day 3: Back and Biceps
1. **Upper Curls (10 to 15 reps)**
2. **Seated Rows (10 to 15 reps)**
3. **Lower Curls (10 to 15 reps)**
4. **Lat Pulls (10 to 15 reps)**

Day 4: Cardio (Repeat 2 or 3 times)
1. **Jump Rope (45 to 90 seconds); rest 10 seconds**
2. **Jump Rope (45 to 90 seconds); rest 10 seconds**

Day 5: Legs
1. **Reverse Lunges (10 to 15 reps)**
2. **Plie Squats (10 to 15 reps)**
3. **Side Lunges (10 to 15 reps)**
4. **Curtsy Squats (10 to 15 reps)**

Day 6: Be Active
Jump in a pool and play water polo.

Day 7: Rest Day

Day 8: Abs and Shoulders
1. **V-Ups (10 to 15 reps)**
2. **Overhead Presses (10 to 15 reps)**
3. **Starfishes (10 to 15 reps)**
4. **Upright Rows (10 to 15 reps)**

Day 9: Cardio (Repeat 2 or 3 times)
1. **Inch Worms (10 to 15 reps)**
2. **Froggers (10 to 15 reps)**
3. **High Knees (10 to 15 reps)**
4. **Inch Worms (10 to 15 reps)**

Day 10: Chest and Triceps
1. **Chest Presses (10 to 15 reps)**
2. **Triceps Kickbacks (10 to 15 reps)**
3. **Push-Ups (10 to 15 reps)**
4. **Skull Crushers (10 to 15 reps)**

Day 11: Cardio (Repeat 2 or 3 times)
1. **Surrenders (10 to 15 reps)**
2. **Jumping Jacks (20 to 30 reps)**
3. **Kickboxing Kicks (10 to 15 reps)**
4. **Jumping Jacks (20 to 30 reps)**

Day 12: Back and Biceps
1. **Concentration Curls (10 to 15 reps)**
2. **Supermans (10 to 15 reps)**
3. **Biceps Curls (10 to 15 reps)**
4. **Renegade Rows (10 to 15 reps)**

Day 13: Be Active
Go for a swim.

Day 14: Rest Day

Day 15: Legs

1. **Bridges** (10 to 15 reps, each with a 30-second hold at the top of the movement)
2. **Bulgarian Lunges** (10 to 15 reps)
3. **Step-Ups** (10 to 15 reps)
4. **Donkey Kicks** (10 to 15 reps)

Day 16: Cardio (Repeat 2 or 3 times)

1. **Burpees** (10 to 15 reps)
2. **Windmills** (20 to 30 reps)
3. **High Knees** (10 to 15 reps)
4. **Windmills** (20 to 30 reps)

Day 17: Abs and Shoulders

1. **Roll-Ups** (10 to 15 reps)
2. **Shoulder Shrugs** (10 to 15 reps)
3. **Mason Twists** (10 to 15 reps)
4. **T Raises** (10 to 15 reps)

Day 18: Cardio (Repeat 2 or 3 times)

1. **Heismans** (30 to 60 seconds)
2. **Inch Worms** (10 to 15 reps)
3. **Squat Thrusts** (10 to 15 reps)
4. **Heismans** (30 to 60 seconds)

Day 19: Chest and Triceps

1. **Incline Push-Ups** (10 to 15 reps)
2. **Diamond Push-Ups** (10 to 15 reps)
3. **Chest Flies** (10 to 15 reps)
4. **Skull Crushers** (10 to 15 reps)

Day 20: Be Active

Play volleyball.

Day 21: Rest Day

Day 22: Back and Biceps

1. **7s** (3 sets)
2. **Bent-Over Flies** (10 to 15 reps)
3. **Hammer Curls** (10 to 15 reps)
4. **Bent-Over Rows** (10 to 15 reps)

Day 23: Cardio (Repeat 2 or 3 times)

1. **Burpees** (10 to 15 reps)
2. **Windmills** (20 to 30 reps)
3. **Kickboxing Kicks** (20 to 30 reps)
4. **Froggers** (10 to 15 reps)

Day 24: Legs

1. **Deadlifts** (10 to 15 reps)
2. **Side Lunges** (10 to 15 reps)
3. **Donkey Kicks** (10 to 15 reps)
4. **Curtsy Lunges** (10 to 15 reps)

Day 25: Cardio (Repeat 2 or 3 times)

1. **Jumping Jacks** (20 to 30 reps)
2. **Inch Worms** (10 to 15 reps)
3. **High Knees** (10 to 15 reps)
4. **Jumping Jacks** (20 to 30 reps)

Day 26: Abs and Shoulders

1. **Criss Crosses** (10 to 15 reps)
2. **Pike Push-Ups** (10 to 15 reps)
3. **Trunk Rotations** (20 to 30 reps)
4. **Milk Pours** (10 to 15 reps)

Day 27: Be Active

Day 28: Rest Day

Day 29: Chest and Triceps

1. **Chest Presses** (10 to 15 reps)
2. **Triceps Dips** (10 to 15 reps)
3. **Incline Push-Ups** (10 to 15 reps)
4. **Triceps Overhead Extensions** (10 to 15 reps)

Day 30: Cardio (Repeat 2 or 3 times)

1. **Jump Rope** (45 to 90 seconds); rest 10 seconds
2. **Jump Rope** (45 to 90 seconds); rest 10 seconds

Day 31: Back and Biceps

1. **Lower Curls** (10 to 15 reps)
2. **Renegade Rows** (10 to o15 reps)
3. **Upper Curls** (10 to 15 reps)
4. **Supermans** (10 to 15 reps)

25. ACTION-PACKED AUGUST

Summer's almost over, but the weather is still rocking. Exercise outside to enjoy the beautiful days and evenings.

Note: While the workout plans here indicate the last two days of the week for play and rest, respectively, adjust your workouts as needed so those days fall on weekends if it is most convenient for your schedule. You'll need light dumbbells and a jump rope to complete many of the exercises. For exercises performed on both the right and left side of the body, like lunges, do the number of reps indicated on both sides before continuing. If you don't know how to do an exercise, go to www.maybeiwill.com/challengesbook for instructions.

Day 1: Legs
1. **Bridges (10 to 15 reps, each with a 30-second hold at the top of the movement)**
2. **Step-Ups (10 to 15 reps)**
3. **Fire Hydrants (10 to 15 reps)**
4. **Reverse Lunges (10 to 15 reps)**

Day 2: Cardio (Repeat 2 or 3 times)
1. **Inch Worms (10 to 15 reps)**
2. **Jumping Lunges (10 to 15 reps)**
3. **Inch Worms (10 to 15 reps)**
4. **Jump Squats (10 to 15 reps)**

Day 3: Chest and Triceps
1. **Chest Flies (10 to 15 reps)**
2. **Triceps Kickbacks (10 to 15 reps)**
3. **Push-Ups (10 to 15 reps)**
4. **Skull Crushers (10 to 15 reps)**

Day 4: Cardio (Repeat 2 or 3 times)
1. **High Knees (10 to 15 reps)**
2. **Kickboxing Kicks (20 to 30 reps)**
3. **Squat Thrusts (10 to 15 reps)**
4. **Windmills (20 to 30 reps)**

Day 5: Back and Biceps
1. **Hammer Curls (10 to 15 reps)**
2. **Lat Pulls (10 to 15 reps)**
3. **Concentration Curls (10 to 15 reps)**
4. **Bent-Over Flies (10 to 15 reps)**

Day 6: Be Active
Go paddle boarding.

Day 7: Rest Day

Day 8: Legs
1. **Reverse Lunges (10 to 15 reps)**
2. **Squats (10 to 15 reps)**
3. **Walking Lunges (10 to 15 reps)**
4. **Sumo Squats (10 to 15 reps)**

Day 9: Cardio (Repeat 2 or 3 times)
1. **Jumping Jacks (45 to 90 seconds); rest 10 seconds**
2. **Jumping Jacks (45 to 90 seconds); rest 10 seconds**

Day 10: Abs and Shoulders
1. **Mason Twists (10 to 15 reps)**
2. **Weighted Punches (10 to 15 reps)**
3. **V-Ups (10 to 15 reps)**
4. **T Raises (10 to 15 reps)**

Day 11: Cardio (Repeat 2 or 3 times)
1. **Surrenders (10 to 15 reps)**
2. **Inch Worms (10 to 15 reps)**
3. **Windmills (20 to 30 reps)**
4. **Four Squares (10 to 15 reps)**

Day 12: Chest and Triceps
1. **Chest Flies (10 to 15 reps)**
2. **Overhead Triceps Extension Dips (10 to 15 reps)**
3. **Incline Push-Ups (10 to 15 reps)**
4. **Triceps Dips (10 to 15 reps)**

Day 13: Be Active
Take a walk after dinner.

Day 14: Rest Day

Day 15: Back and Biceps
1. 7s (3 sets)
2. Supermans (10 to 15 reps)
3. W Curls (10 to 15 reps)
4. Renegade Rows (10 to 15 reps)

Day 16: Cardio (Repeat 2 or 3 times)
1. Jump Rope (45 to 90 seconds); rest 10 seconds
2. Jump Rope (45 to 90 seconds); rest 10 seconds

Day 17: Legs
1. Donkey Kicks (10 to 15 reps)
2. Fire Hydrants (10 to 15 reps)
3. Leg Raises (10 to 15 reps)
4. Bridges (10 to 15 reps, each with a 30-second hold at the top of the movement)

Day 18: Cardio
1. Jumping Jacks (20 to 30 reps)
2. Kickboxing Kicks (10 to 15 reps)
3. Burpees (10 to 15 reps)
4. Windmills (20 to 30 reps)

Day 19: Abs and Shoulders
1. Plank (45 to 90 seconds)
2. Overhead Presses (10 to 15 reps)
3. Roll-Ups (10 to 15 reps)
4. V Raises (10 to 15 reps)

Day 20: Be Active
Go kayaking or canoeing.

Day 21: Rest Day

Day 22: Chest and Triceps
1. Chest Flies (10 to 15 reps)
2. Diamond Push-Ups (10 to 15 reps)
3. Decline Push-Ups (10 to 15 reps)
4. Triceps Kickbacks (10 to 15 reps)

Day 23: Cardio (Repeat 2 or 3 times)
1. Four Corners (10 to 15 reps)
2. Skaters (10 to 15 reps)
3. Jumping Jacks (20 to 30 reps)
4. Inch Worms (10 to 15 reps)

Day 24: Back and Biceps
1. Hammer Curls (10 to 15 reps)
2. Seated Rows (10 to 15 reps)
3. W Curls (10 to 15 reps)
4. Lat Pulls (10 to 15 reps)

Day 25: Cardio (Repeat 2 or 3 times)
1. Kickboxing Kicks (10 to 15 reps)
2. High Knees (10 to 15 reps)
3. Windmills (20 to 30 reps)
4. Squat Thrusts (10 to 15 reps)

Day 26: Legs
1. Deadlifts (10 to 15 reps)
2. Step-Ups (10 to 15 reps)
3. Side Lunges (10 to 15 reps)
4. Sumo Squats (10 to 15 reps)

Day 27: Be Active
Try line dancing.

Day 28: Rest Day

Day 29: Abs and Shoulders
1. Swimmers (100 counts)
2. Pike Push-Ups (10 to 15 reps)
3. Mason Twists (10 to 15 reps)
4. Weighted Arm Circles (10 to 15 reps)

Day 30: Cardio (Repeat 2 or 3 times)
1. Burpees (45 to 90 seconds); rest 10 seconds
2. Burpees (45 to 90 seconds); rest 10 seconds

Day 31: Chest and Triceps
1. Chest Presses (10 to 15 reps)
2. Triceps Kickbacks (10 to 15 reps)
3. Push-Ups (10 to 15 reps)
4. Skull Crushers (10 to 15 reps)

26. SASSY SEPTEMBER

As the seasons change, reevaluate and refocus your goals.

Note: While the workout plans here indicate the last two days of the week for play and rest, respectively, adjust your workouts as needed so those days fall on weekends if it is most convenient for your schedule. You'll need light dumbbells and a jump rope to complete many of the exercises. For exercises performed on both the right and left side of the body, like lunges, do the number of reps indicated on both sides before continuing. If you don't know how to do an exercise, go to www.maybeiwill.com/challengesbook for instructions.

Day 1: Back and Biceps
1. **Concentration Curls (10 to 15 reps)**
2. **Supermans (10 to 15 reps)**
3. **Alternating Biceps Curls (10 to 15 reps)**
4. **Renegade Rows (10 to 15 reps)**

Day 2: Cardio (Repeat 2 or 3 times)
1. **Surrenders (10 to 15 reps)**
2. **High Knees (10 to 15 reps)**
3. **Inch Worms (10 to 15 reps)**
4. **Mountain Climbers (10 to 15 reps)**

Day 3: Legs
1. **Squats (10 to 15 reps)**
2. **Bulgarian Lunges (10 to 15 reps)**
3. **Curtsy Lunges (10 to 15 reps)**
4. **Sumo Squats (10 to 15 reps)**

Day 4: Cardio (Repeat 2 or 3 times)
1. **Kickboxing Kicks (10 to 15 reps)**
2. **Wide Arm Circles (10 to 15 reps)**
3. **Surrenders (10 to 15 reps)**
4. **Froggers (10 to 15 reps)**

Day 5: Abs and Shoulders
1. **Plank (45 to 90 seconds)**
2. **Shoulder Shrugs (10 to 15 reps)**
3. **Swimmers (100 counts)**
4. **Milk Pours (10 to 15 reps)**

Day 6: Be Active
Play a game of football.

Day 7: Rest Day

Day 8: Chest and Triceps
1. **Chest Presses (10 to 15 reps)**
2. **Diamond Push-Ups (10 to 15 reps)**
3. **Chest Flies (10 to 15 reps)**
4. **Triceps Dips (10 to 15 reps)**

Day 9: Cardio (Repeat 2 or 3 times)
1. **Jump Rope (45 to 90 seconds); rest 10 seconds**
2. **Jumping Jacks (45 to 90 seconds); rest 10 seconds**

Day 10: Back and Biceps
1. **7s (3 sets)**
2. **Bent-Over Rows (10 to 15 reps)**
3. **Hammer Curls (10 to 15 reps)**
4. **Bent-Over Flies (10 to 15 reps)**

Day 11: Cardio (Repeat 2 or 3 times)
1. **Froggers (10 to 15 reps)**
2. **Jumping Lunges (10 to 15 reps)**
3. **Inch Worms (10 to 15 reps)**
4. **Froggers (10 to 15 reps)**

Day 12: Legs
1. **Bridges (10 to 15 reps, each with a 30-second hold at the top of the movement)**
2. **Deadlifts (10 to 15 reps)**
3. **Step-Ups (10 to 15 reps)**
4. **Side Lunges (10 to 15 reps)**

Day 13: Be Active
Try a round of disc golf.

Day 14: Rest Day

Day 15: Abs and Shoulders

1. Crunches (20 to 30 reps)
2. T Raises (10 to 15 reps)
3. Criss Crosses (10 to 15 reps)
4. Upright Rows (10 to 15 reps)

Day 16: Cardio (Repeat 2 or 3 times)

1. Jumping Jacks (20 to 30 reps)
2. Windmills (20 to 30 reps)
3. Jumping Jacks (20 to 30 reps)
4. Windmills (20 to 30 reps)

Day 17: Chest and Triceps

1. Incline Push-Ups (10 to 15 reps)
2. Skull Crushers (10 to 15 reps)
3. Chest Presses (10 to 15 reps)
4. Triceps Overhead Presses (10 to 15 reps)

Day 18 : Cardio (Repeat 2 or 3 times)

1. Jumping Lunges (10 to 15 reps)
2. Inch Worms (10 to 15 reps)
3. Jump Squats (10 to 15 reps)
4. Wide Arm Circles (20 to 30 reps)

Day 19: Back and Biceps

1. Hammer Curls (10 to 15 reps)
2. Seated Rows (10 to 15 reps)
3. W Curls (10 to 15 reps)
4. Supermans (10 to 15 reps)

Day 20: Be Active

Play a game of racquetball.

Day 21: Rest Day

Day 22: Leg Day

1. Bridges (10 to 15 reps, each with a 30-second hold at the top of the movement)
2. Deadlifts (10 to 15 reps)
3. Step-Ups (10 to 15 reps)
4. Side Lunges (10 to 15 reps)

Day 23: Cardio (Repeat 2 or 3 times)

1. Froggers (10 to 15 reps)
2. Four Corners (10 to 15 reps)
3. Skaters (10 to 15 reps)
4. High Knees (10 to 15 reps)

Day 24: Abs and Shoulders

1. Weighted Side Bends (10 to 15 reps)
2. Weighted Punches (10 to 15 reps)
3. Roll-Ups (10 to 15 reps)
4. Weighted Arm Circles (10 to 15 reps)

Day 25: Cardio (Repeat 2 or 3 times)

1. Jump Rope (45 to 90 seconds); rest 10 seconds
2. Jump Rope (45 to 90 seconds); rest 10 seconds

Day 26: Chest and Triceps

1. Chest Presses (10 to 15 reps)
2. Skull Crushers (10 to 15 reps)
3. Decline Push-Ups (10 to 15 reps)
4. Overhead Triceps Extensions (10 to 15 reps)

Day 27: Be Active

Go for a hike.

Day 28: Rest Day

Day 29: Back and Biceps

1. Upper Curls (10 to 15 reps)
2. Bent-Over Rows (10 to 15 reps)
3. Lower Curls (10 to 15 reps)
4. Bent-Over Flies (10 to 15 reps)

Day 30: Cardio (Repeat 2 or 3 times)

1. Surrenders (10 to 15 reps)
2. Windmills (20 to 30 reps)
3. Inch Worms (10 to 15 reps)
4. Squat Thrusts (10 to 15 reps)

27. OPPORTUNE OCTOBER

It's getting chilly and Halloween candy is everywhere. Just stay focused on fitness. You got this!

Note: While the workout plans here indicate the last two days of the week for play and rest, respectively, adjust your workouts as needed so those days fall on weekends if it is most convenient for your schedule. You'll need light dumbbells and a jump rope to complete many of the exercises. For exercises performed on both the right and left side of the body, like lunges, do the number of reps indicated on both sides before continuing. If you don't know how to do an exercise, go to www.maybeiwill.com/challengesbook for instructions.

Day 1: Legs
1. **Reverse Lunges (10 to 15 reps)**
2. **Plie Squats (10 to 15 reps)**
3. **Leg Lifts (10 to 15 reps)**
4. **Sumo Squats (10 to 15 reps)**

Day 2: Cardio (Repeat 2 or 3 times)
1. **Burpees (45 to 90 seconds); rest 10 seconds**
2. **Burpees (45 to 90 seconds); rest 10 seconds**

Day 3: Abs and Shoulders
1. **Trunk Rotations (20 to 30 reps)**
2. **Upright Rows (10 to 15 reps)**
3. **V-Ups (10 to 15 reps)**
4. **T Raises (10 to 15 reps)**

Day 4: Cardio (Repeat 2 or 3 times)
1. **Skaters (10 to 15 reps)**
2. **High Knees (10 to 15 reps)**
3. **Kickboxing Kicks (10 to 15 reps)**
4. **Jumping Lunges (10 to 15 reps)**

Day 5: Chest and Triceps
1. **Push-Ups (10 to 15 reps)**
2. **Triceps Dips (10 to 15 reps)**
3. **Chest Flies (10 to 15 reps)**
4. **Skull Crushers (10 to 15 reps)**

Day 6: Be Active
Challenge some friends to a game of touch football.

Day 7: Rest Day

Day 8: Back and Biceps
1. **Alternating Biceps Curls (10 to 15 reps)**
2. **Renegade Rows (10 to 15 reps)**
3. **Hammer Curls (10 to 15 reps)**
4. **Seated Rows (10 to 15 reps)**

Day 9: Cardio (Repeat 2 or 3 times)
1. **High Knees (10 to 15 reps)**
2. **Windmills (20 to 30 reps)**
3. **Jumping Jacks (20 to 30 reps)**
4. **Skaters (10 to 15 reps)**

Day 10: Legs
1. **Donkey Kicks (10 to 15 reps)**
2. **Fire Hydrants (10 to 15 reps)**
3. **Bridges (10 to 15 reps, each with a 30-second hold at the top of the movement)**
4. **Leg Lifts (10 to 15 reps)**

Day 11: Cardio (Repeat 2 or 3 times)
1. **Heismans (45 to 90 seconds); rest 10 seconds**
2. **Heismans (45 to 90 seconds); rest 10 seconds**

Day 12: Abs and Shoulders
1. **Plank (45 to 90 seconds)**
2. **T Raises (10 to 15 reps)**
3. **Plank Dips (10 to 15 reps)**
4. **V Raises (10 to 15 reps)**

Day 13: Be Active
Try your hand at juggling.

Day 14: Rest Day

Day 15: Chest and Triceps
1. **Chest Flies (10 to 15 reps)**
2. **Triceps Kickbacks (10 to 15 reps)**
3. **Incline Push-Ups (10 to 15 reps)**
4. **Overhead Triceps Extensions (10 to 15 reps)**

Day 16: Cardio (Repeat 2 or 3 times)
1. **Skaters (10 to 15 reps)**
2. **Jumping Jacks (10 to 15 reps)**
3. **High Knees (10 to 15 reps)**
4. **Froggers (10 to 15 reps)**

Day 17: Back and Biceps

1. Concentration Curls (10 to 15 reps)
2. Renegade Rows (10 to 15 reps)
3. Hammer Curls (10 to 15 reps)
4. Lat Pulls (10 to 15 reps)

Day 18: Cardio (Repeat 2 or 3 times)

1. Inch Worms (10 to 15 reps)
2. Windmills (20 to 30 reps)
3. Jumping Jacks (20 to 30 reps)
4. Inch Worms (10 to 15 reps)

Day 19: Legs

1. Bulgarian Lunges (10 to 15 reps)
2. Plie Squats (10 to 15 reps)
3. Calf Raises (20 reps, each with a 5- to 10-second hold at the top of the movement)
4. Lunges (10 to 15 reps)

Day 20: Be Active

Spend the day raking leaves--extra points for running and jumping into them and having to rake them again.

Day 21: Rest Day

Day 22: Abs and Shoulders

1. Swimmers (100 counts)
2. Milk Pours (10 to 15 reps)
3. Starfishes (10 to 15 reps)
4. Overhead Presses (10 to 15 reps)

Day 23: Cardio (Repeat 2 or 3 times)

1. Jump Rope (45 to 90 seconds); rest 10 seconds
2. Jump Rope (45 to 90 seconds); rest 10 seconds

Day 24: Chest and Triceps

1. Decline Push-Ups (10 to 15 reps)
2. Triceps Kickbacks (10 to 15 reps)
3. Chest Presses (10 to 15 reps)
4. Triceps Dips (10 to 15 reps)

Day 25: Cardio (Repeat 2 or 3 times)

1. Jumping Lunges (10 to 15 reps)
2. Windmills (20 to 30 reps)
3. Jump Squats (10 to 15 reps)
4. Windmills (20 to 30 reps)

Day 26: Back and Biceps

1. 7s (3 sets)
2. Bent-Over Rows (10 to 15 reps)
3. Alternating Biceps Curls (10 to 15 reps)
4. Supermans (10 to 15 reps)

Day 27: Be Active

Check out a corn maze.

Day 28: Rest Day

Day 29:

Do stair runs (or sprints if you don't have access to stairs). Go full effort for 45 seconds up and down followed by a 1-minute walking cooldown. Repeat 3 to 5 times.

Day 30: Leg Day

1. Deadlifts (10 to 15 reps)
2. Curtsy Lunges (10 to 15 reps)
3. Bridges (10 to 15 reps, each with a 30-second hold at the top of the movement)
4. Side Lunges (10 to 15 reps)

Day 31: Cardio (Repeat 2 or 3 times)

1. Burpees (45 to 90 seconds); rest 10 seconds
2. Burpees (45 to 90 seconds); rest 10 seconds

28. NOURISHING NOVEMBER

November is a great time to nourish your body by exercising. Take time to offer sincere gratitude to your body for how amazing it is!

Note: While the workout plans here indicate the last two days of the week for play and rest, respectively, adjust your workouts as needed so those days fall on weekends if it is most convenient for your schedule. You'll need light dumbbells and a jump rope to complete many of the exercises. For exercises performed on both the right and left side of the body, like lunges, do the number of reps indicated on both sides before continuing. If you don't know how to do an exercise, go to www.maybeiwill.com/challengesbook for instructions.

Day 1: Abs and Shoulders
1. **Ab Rotations (20 to 30 reps)**
2. **Upright Rows (10 to 15 reps)**
3. **Mason Twists (10 to 15 reps)**
4. **Pike Push-Ups (10 to 15 reps)**

Day 2: Cardio (Repeat 2 or 3 times)
1. **Surrenders (10 to 15 reps)**
2. **Wide Arm Circles (20 to 30 reps)**
3. **Skaters (10 to 15 reps)**
4. **Kickboxing Kicks (10 to 15 reps)**

Day 3: Chest to Triceps
1. **Chest Presses (10 to 15 reps)**
2. **Skull Crushers (10 to 15 reps)**
3. **Chest Flies (10 to 15 reps)**
4. **Diamond Push-Ups (10 to 15 reps)**

Day 4: Cardio
1. **Inch Worms (10 to 15 reps)**
2. **Jumping Lunges (10 to 15 reps)**
3. **Windmills (20 to 30 reps)**
4. **Jump Squats (10 to 15 reps)**

Day 5: Back and Biceps
1. **Hammer Curls (10 to 15 reps)**
2. **Supermans (10 to 15 reps)**
3. **Concentration Curls (10 to 15 reps)**
4. **Seated Rows (10 to 15 reps)**

Day 6: Be Active
Challenge some friends to a game of touch football.

Day 7: Rest Day

Day 8: Legs
1. **Donkey Kicks (10 to 15 reps)**
2. **Fire Hydrants (10 to 15 reps)**
3. **Side Lunges (10 to 15 reps)**
4. **Glute Bridges (10 to 15 reps)**

Day 9: Cardio (Repeat 2 or 3 times)
1. **Jumping Jacks (45 to 90 seconds); rest 10 seconds**
2. **Jumping Jacks (45 to 90 seconds); rest 10 seconds**

Day 10: Abs and Shoulders
1. **V-Ups (10 to 15 reps)**
2. **Milk Pours (10 to 15 reps)**
3. **Criss Crosses (10 to 15 reps)**
4. **Overhead Presses (10 to 15 reps)**

Day 11: Cardio (Repeat 2 or 3 times)
1. **Skaters (10 to 15 reps)**
2. **Froggers (10 to 15 reps)**
3. **Skaters (10 to 15 reps)**
4. **Froggers (10 to 15 reps)**

Day 12: Chest and Triceps
1. **Incline Push-Ups (10 to 15 reps)**
2. **Triceps Dips (10 to 15 reps)**
3. **Chest Presses (10 to 15 reps)**
4. **Skull Crushers (10 to 15 reps)**

Day 13: Be Active
Challenge a friend to a game of ping-pong.

Day 14: Rest Day

Day 15: Back and Biceps

1. **7s (3 sets)**
2. **Bent-Over Rows (10 to 15 reps)**
3. **Hammer Curls (10 to 15 reps)**
4. **Bent-Over Flies (10 to 15 reps)**

Day 16: Cardio (Repeat 2 or 3 times)

1. **Jumping Jacks (20 to 30 reps)**
2. **Windmills (20 to 30 reps)**
3. **High Knees (10 to 15 reps)**
4. **Jumping Jacks (20 to 30 reps)**

Day 17: Legs

1. **Deadlifts (10 to 15 reps)**
2. **Step-Ups (10 to 15 reps)**
3. **Sumo Squats (10 to 15 reps)**
4. **Curtsy Lunges (10 to 15 reps)**

Day 18: Cardio (Repeat 2 or 3 times)

1. **Four Corners (10 to 15 reps)**
2. **Skaters (10 to 15 reps)**
3. **Inch Worms (10 to 15 reps)**
4. **Wide Arm Circles (20 to 30 reps)**

Day 19: Abs and Shoulders

1. **Swimmers (100 counts)**
2. **T Raises (10 to 15 reps)**
3. **Starfishes (10 to 15 reps)**
4. **V Raises (10 to 15 reps)**

Day 20: Be Active

Find a service project to volunteer for.

Day 21: Rest Day

Day 22: Chest and Triceps

1. **Chest Flies (10 to 15 reps)**
2. **Overhead Triceps Extensions (10 to 15 reps)**
3. **Decline Push-Ups (10 to 15 reps)**
4. **Triceps Kickbacks (10 to 15 reps)**

Day 23: Cardio (Repeat 2 or 3 times)

1. **Jump Rope (45 to 90 seconds); rest 10 seconds**
2. **Jump Rope (45 to 90 seconds); rest 10 seconds**

Day 24: Back and Biceps

1. **Alternating Biceps Curls (10 to 15 reps)**
2. **Supermans (10 to 15 reps)**
3. **Biceps Curls (10 to 15 reps)**
4. **Lat Pulls (10 to 15 reps)**

Day 25: Cardio (Repeat 2 or 3 times)

1. **Skaters (10 to 15 reps)**
2. **Froggers (10 to 15 reps)**
3. **Kickboxing Kicks (10 to 15 reps)**
4. **High Knees (10 to 15 reps)**

Day 26: Leg Day

1. **Plie Squats (10 to 15 reps)**
2. **Reverse Lunges (10 to 15 reps)**
3. **Sumo Squats (10 to 15 reps)**
4. **Bulgarian Lunges (10 to 15 reps)**

Day 27: Be Active

Take a long walk and think about all the things you're grateful for.

Day 28: Rest Day

Day 29: Abs and Shoulders

1. **Plank Dips (10 to 15 reps)**
2. **Shoulder Shrugs (10 to 15 reps)**
3. **Roll-Ups (10 to 15 reps)**
4. **Weighted Punches (10 to 15 reps)**

Day 30: Cardio (Repeat 2 or 3 times)

1. **Jumping Lunges (10 to 15 reps)**
2. **Inch Worms (10 to 15 reps)**
3. **Burpees (10 to 15 reps)**
4. **Windmills (20 to 30 reps)**

29. DEDICATED DECEMBER

The holidays are in full swing and you have a million things to do. You may be busy and stressed, but dedicating time each day to working out will help reduce stress and keep your energy up.

Note: While the workout plans here indicate the last two days of the week for play and rest, respectively, adjust your workouts as needed so those days fall on weekends if it is most convenient for your schedule. You'll need light dumbbells and a jump rope to complete many of the exercises. For exercises performed on both the right and left side of the body, like lunges, do the number of reps indicated on both sides before continuing. If you don't know how to do an exercise, go to www.maybeiwill.com/challengesbook for instructions.

Day 1: Chest and Triceps
1. **Push-Ups (10 to 15 reps)**
2. **Skull Crushers (10 to 15 reps)**
3. **Chest Presses (10 to 15 reps)**
4. **Diamond Push-Ups (10 to 15 reps)**

Day 2: Cardio (Repeat 2 or 3 times)
1. **Froggers (10 to 15 reps)**
2. **Skaters (10 to 15 reps)**
3. **Wide Arm Circles (20 to 30 reps)**
4. **Jumping Jacks (20 to 30 reps)**

Day 3: Back and Biceps
1. **Hammer Curls (10 to 15 reps)**
2. **Renegade Rows (10 to 15 reps)**
3. **W Curls (10 to 15 reps)**
4. **Seated Rows (10 to 15 reps)**

Day 4: Cardio (Repeat 2 or 3 times)
1. **Jump Rope (45 to 90 seconds); rest 10 seconds**
2. **Jump Rope (45 to 90 seconds); rest 10 seconds**

Day 5: Leg Day
1. **Donkey Kicks (10 to 15 reps)**
2. **Fire Hydrants (10 to 15 reps)**
3. **Leg Raises (10 to 15 reps)**
4. **Bridges (10 to 15 reps, each with a 30-second hold at the top of the movement)**

Day 6: Be Active
Go ice skating.

Day 7: Rest Day

Day 8: Abs and Shoulders
1. **Mason Twists (10 to 15 reps)**
2. **Upright Rows (10 to 15 reps)**
3. **V-Ups (10 to 15 reps)**
4. **T Raises (10 to 15 reps)**

Day 9: Cardio (Repeat 2 or 3 times)
1. **Jumping Lunges (10 to 15 reps)**
2. **Inch Worms (10 to 15 reps)**
3. **Jump Squats (10 to 15 reps)**
4. **Windmills (20 to 30 reps)**

Day 10: Chest and Triceps
1. **Push-Ups (10 to 15 reps)**
2. **Skull Crushers (10 to 15 reps)**
3. **Chest Flies (10 to 15 reps)**
4. **Overhead Triceps Extensions (10 to 15 reps)**

Day 11: Cardio (Repeat 2 or 3 times)
1. **Crab Walks (45 to 90 seconds)**
2. **Windmills (20 to 30 reps)**
3. **Bear Walks (45 to 90 seconds)**
4. **Windmills (20 to 30 reps)**

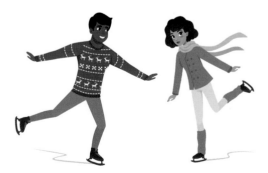

Day 12: Back and Biceps

1. **Alternating Curls (10 to 15 reps)**
2. **Supermans (10 to 15 reps)**
3. **Biceps Curls (10 to 15 reps)**
4. **Seated Rows (10 to 15 reps)**

Day 13: Be Active

Go holiday shopping.

Day 14: Rest Day

Day 15: Legs

1. **Side Lunges (10 to 15 reps)**
2. **Reverse Lunges (10 to 15 reps)**
3. **Curtsy Lunges (10 to 15 reps)**
4. **Bulgarian Lunges (10 to 15 reps)**

Day 16: Cardio (Repeat 2 or 3 times)

1. **Froggers (10 to 15 reps)**
2. **Inch Worms (10 to 15 reps)**
3. **Burpees (10 to 15 reps)**
4. **Skaters (10 to 15 reps)**

Day 17: Abs and Shoulders

1. **Sit-Ups (20 to 30 reps)**
2. **Milk Pours (10 to 15 reps)**
3. **Plank (45 to 90 seconds)**
4. **Shoulder Shrugs (10 to 15 reps)**

Day 18: Cardio (Repeat 2 or 3 times)

1. **Jump Rope (45 to 90 seconds); rest 10 seconds**
2. **Jump Rope (45 to 90 seconds); rest 10 seconds**

Day 19: Chest and Triceps

1. **Chest Presses (10 to 15 reps)**
2. **Diamond Push-Ups (10 to 15 reps)**
3. **Chest Flies (10 to 15 reps)**
4. **Triceps Dips (10 to 15 reps)**

Day 20: Be Active

Have a snowball fight!

Day 21: Rest Day

Day 22: Back and Biceps

1. **7s (3 sets)**
2. **Renegade Rows (10 to 15 reps)**
3. **Hammer Curls (10 to 15 reps)**
4. **Lat Pulls (10 to 15 reps)**

Day 23: Cardio

1. **Heismans (45 to 90 seconds)**
2. **Windmills (20 to 30 reps)**
3. **Heismans (45 to 90 seconds)**
4. **Windmills (20 to 30 reps)**

Day 24: Legs (Repeat 2 or 3 times)

1. **Step-Ups (10 to 15 reps)**
2. **Deadlifts (10 to 15 reps)**
3. **Sumo Squats (10 to 15 reps)**
4. **Bridges (10 to 15 reps, each with a 30-second hold at the top)**

Day 25: Cardio (Repeat 2 or 3 times)

1. **Jumping Jacks (20 to 30 reps)**
2. **Inch Worms (10 to 15 reps)**
3. **Jumping Jacks (20 to 30 reps)**
4. **Inch Worms (10 to 15 reps)**

Day 26: Be Active

Organize your house for the new year.

Day 27: Rest Day

Day 28: Abs and Shoulders

1. **Trunk Rotations (20 to 30 reps)**
2. **T Raises (10 to 15 reps)**
3. **Mason Twists (10 to 15 reps)**
4. **V Raises (10 to 15 reps)**

Day 29: Cardio (Repeat 2 or 3 times)

1. **Jumping Lunges (10 to 15 reps)**
2. **Skaters (10 to 15 reps)**
3. **Jump Squats (10 to 15 reps)**
4. **Froggers (10 to 15 reps)**

Day 30: Chest and Triceps

1. **Push-Ups (10 to 15 reps)**
2. **Overhead Triceps Extensions (10 to 15 reps)**
3. **Chest Presses (10 to 15 reps)**
4. **Diamond Push-Ups (10 to 15 reps)**

Day 31: Cardio (Repeat 2 or 3 times)

1. **Jump Rope (45 to 90 seconds); rest 10 seconds**
2. **Jump Rope (45 to 90 seconds); rest 10 seconds**

30. PUMP UP WITH PUSH-UPS

People will think I am crazy by admitting this, but push-ups are by far my favorite exercise. I *love* doing push-ups!

Push-ups, like planks, work your entire body and really help to tone and sculpt your arms.

Here is a pro tip for my female friends: Keep your arm stance narrow. *Do not* do wide push-ups. Wide push-ups are not a girl's friend as they can add bulk throughout the shoulders where we gals really do no not want to be any wider. So ladies, keep your stance narrow, and guys, by all means keep your push-ups wide!

For this challenge you'll be doing push-ups every day for 30 days. On the first day do as many as you are able without going too crazy, and this will be your baseline. Increase by one or two push-ups every few days.

FOR EXAMPLE:

Day 1:	5 Push-Ups
Days 2–3:	5 Push-Ups
Days 4–6:	6 Push-Ups
Days 7–10:	7 Push-Ups

Listen to your body and do as many as you can daily. If you need to do modified push-ups that's fine, but try to do at least one on your toes every day, adding more as you are able. Remember, you are *way stronger than you think you are!*

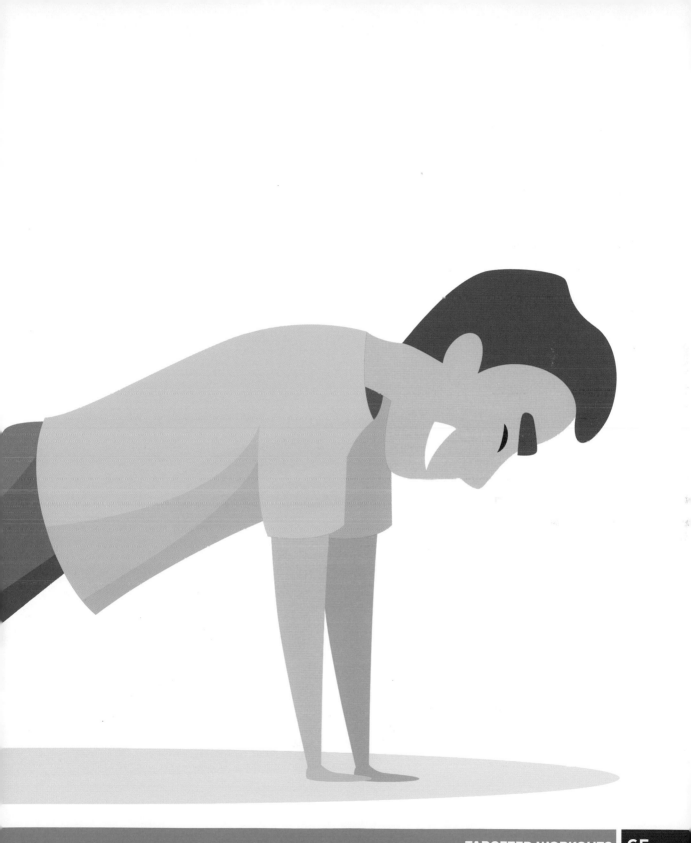

31. DO A FAMILY PUSH-UPS CHALLENGE

My kids are my everything. Each of them came bounding into this world with their very own personality and purpose. They astound me all the time with how truly amazing and also how *very* different they are.

My husband and I had dreams of having kids that were athletic and super into sports. I love my kids dearly, but that is none of their passions. So although my kids are not active in any team sports, except my oldest girl who surprised us all and fell in love with wrestling, we still love to find fun ways to keep them active.

One year we decided that we were going to challenge the kids to do 10 push-ups every night. We started out strong, all of us lining up every night to do our 10 push-ups together as a family. We lasted a few months and it was so much fun!

The idea here is to get in the habit of supporting active movement while enjoying some one-on-one time with the kids. Our seven-year-old's form is lacking but we have fun helping her to learn how to work toward a proper push-up!

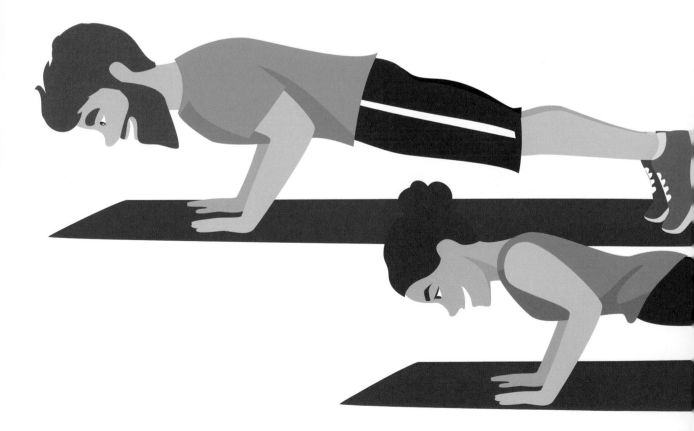

For this challenge, gather the family and commit to doing 10 push-ups each day for 30 days. If it works well for your family, keep it going! We may have petered out after 3 months, but we still try to get our push-ups in more often than not.

Some of your children, and maybe even you, will need to start with modified push-ups and that is totally OK! Begin wherever you are and try to become a little stronger every day.

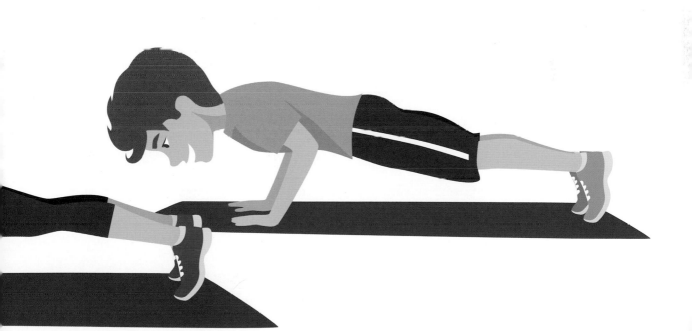

32. SAY YES TO SQUATS

Squats are ideal to build and tone your booty. This challenge is easy to do every day for 30 days, and you'll be thrilled with the improvement to your butt and legs.

To do a basic squat, stand with your feet shoulder-width apart. Keeping your spine straight and your abs tight, slowly lower your body. Do not let your knees pass in front of your toes. Slowly return to the starting position.

MIX IT UP WITH THESE SQUAT VARIATIONS:

» **Curtsy squat.** Stand upright with your arms facing out. As you lower your body lift one foot off the floor and cross it behind the other leg. Keep your arms facing out and slowly lower your body until your hips are in a basic squat position. Drive up through your standing leg and repeat on both sides.

» **Sumo squat.** Stand in a wide stance with your toes pointing out. Bend your knees to lower until your thighs are parallel with the floor. Straighten your legs to stand, squeezing your glutes at the top.

» **Jump squat.** Do a basic squat. At the bottom, engage your core and jump up explosively. When you land, lower your body back into the squat position to complete one rep. Be as gentle on your landing as possible.

» **Plie squat.** Stand in a wide stance with your toes slightly turned out. Bend at the knees into a slight squat, lifting one heel so you're on your toes. Keep the other foot flat on the ground. Lower your butt a few inches toward the ground while keeping your chest up and spine straight.

» **Single-leg squat.** Stand on one foot with your other leg bent at the knee. You can also make it easier by holding both arms out in front of you during the exercise for balance. Once you're balanced on one leg, squat down as low as you can without losing your form or toppling over. Hold on to the back of a chair for balance, if needed.

» **Pistol squat.** This advanced single-leg squat has the raised leg extended straight out in front while you squat.

On Day 1 of the challenge, do as many squats as you can without going too crazy. This will be your baseline. Every day after that, add one more squat.

FOR EXAMPLE:

Day 1:	10 Squats
Day 2:	11 Squats
Day 3:	12 Squats
Day 4:	13 Squats

You get the idea. Now get to squatting! Your booty will thank you.

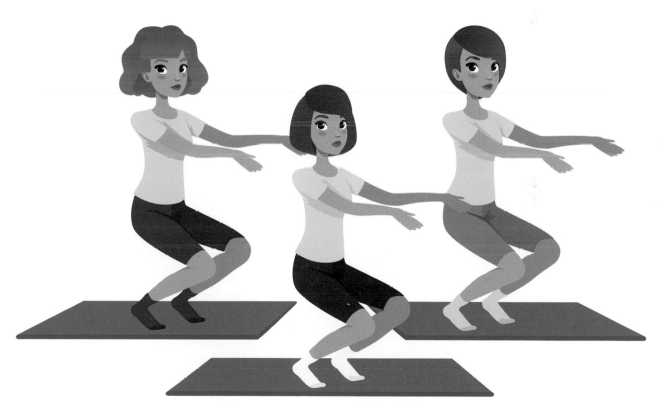

33. LEARN TO LOVE LUNGES

Lunges are a great way to tone your entire lower half. This simple movement targets not only the glutes, but the quadriceps and hamstrings. You'll see improvement in balance, core strength, and hip flexibility, making lunges a pretty powerful tool.

To do a static lunge, step forward into a split stance and lower your body until the front thigh and back shin are parallel to the ground without touching the ground. Return to the standing position and repeat on the other side.

MIX THINGS UP WITH THESE LUNGE VARIATIONS:

» **Front lunge.** Stand with your feet hip-width apart, engage your core, and take a big step forward. Keeping your upper body upright, activate your glutes and bend your front knee to lower your body until the back knee lightly taps the floor. Drive your front heel into the floor to return to the starting position. Repeat on the other side.

» **Reverse lunge.** Stand with your feet hip-width apart, engage your core, and take a big step backward. Keeping your upper body upright, activate your glutes and bend your front knee to lower your body until the back knee lightly taps the floor. Drive your front heel into the floor to return to the starting position. Repeat on the other side.

» **Side lunge.** Stand with your feet slightly wider than shoulder-distance apart and toes pointed forward. Shift your body weight to one leg. Bend one knee to 90-degree angle, keeping the other leg straight. Press your glutes back behind you. Return to center and switch sides.

» **Walking lunge.** Do a front lunge with alternating legs, moving forward with each lunge.

» **Jumping lunge.** This is a walking lunge with a jump between each lunge.

» **Clock lunge.** Do a forward lunge, side lunge, and a backward lunge.

» **Curtsy lunge.** Start from standing, and step your left leg behind and to the right so your thighs cross, bending both knees as if you were curtsying.

On Day 1 of the challenge, do as many lunges as you can without going too crazy. This will be your baseline. Every day after that, add one more lunge.

EXAMPLE:

Day 1:	10 Front Lunges
Day 2:	11 Reverse Lunges
Day 3:	12 Side Lunges
Day 4:	13 Curtsy Lunges

Note: To complete one full repetition, do one lunge on the right, then one on the left.

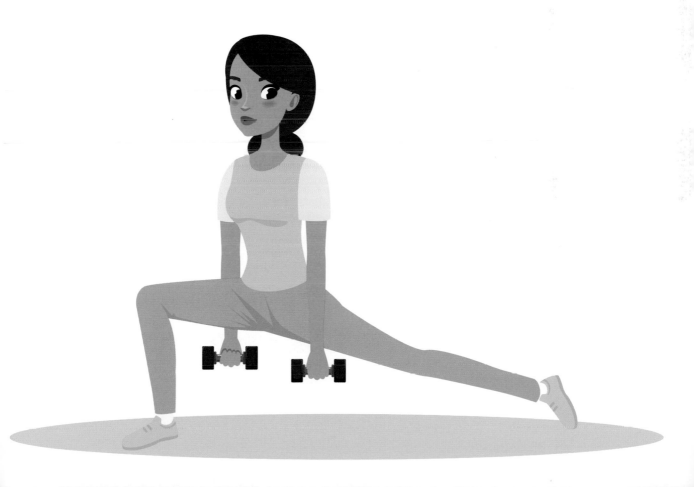

34. PLANK EVERY DAY

Planks are a magical exercise because they are able to target so many muscles groups all at once. So if you commit to this challenge and plank every day for 30 days, you will notice a difference in your fitness.

Most 30-day plank challenges are super tough because while they start out easy at 20 seconds, they quickly amp up to 5 minutes. Five minutes, unless you are already in crazy good shape, is a *long* time to hold a plank.

This challenge is designed to suit all fitness levels and will help you to build your core strength without leaving you feeling defeated.

Day 1:	20 seconds	**Day 17:**	40 seconds
Day 2:	20 seconds	**Day 18:**	40 seconds
Day 3:	25 seconds	**Day 19:**	40 seconds
Day 4:	25 seconds	**Day 20:**	40 seconds
Day 5:	25 seconds	**Day 21:**	40 seconds
Day 6:	25 seconds	**Day 22:**	45 seconds
Day 7:	30 seconds	**Day 23:**	45 seconds
Day 8:	30 seconds	**Day 24:**	45 seconds
Day 9:	30 seconds	**Day 25:**	50 seconds
Day 10:	30 seconds	**Day 26:**	50 seconds
Day 11:	30 seconds	**Day 27:**	55 seconds
Day 12:	35 seconds	**Day 28:**	55 seconds
Day 13:	35 seconds	**Day 29:**	60 seconds
Day 14:	35 seconds	**Day 30:**	60 seconds
Day 15:	35 seconds		
Day 16:	35 seconds		

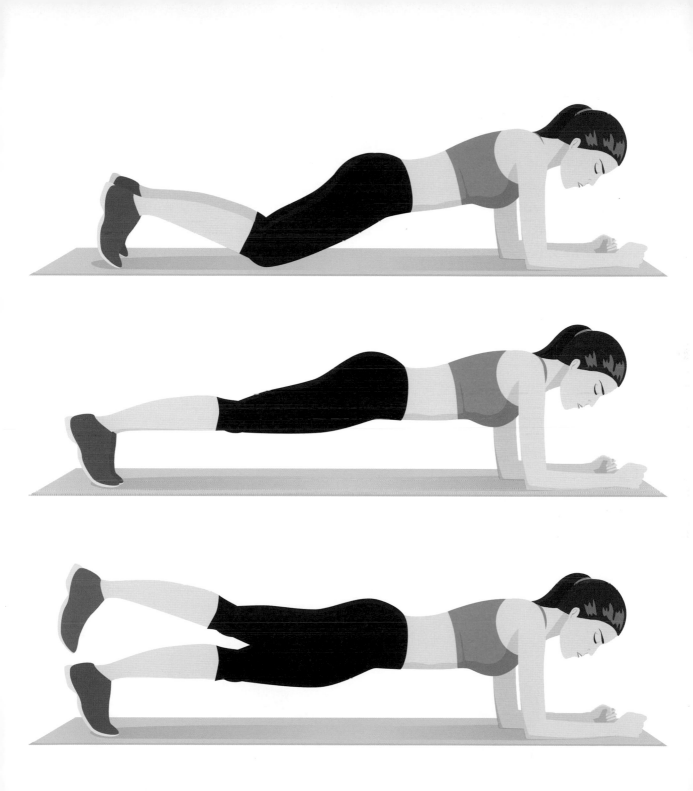

35. SCULPT YOUR ARMS

There is one single exercise that I absolutely give full credit to for my sculpted arms: walkouts. Even when I'm training for a race or another big event, I do not deter from this amazing toning exercise that doesn't require a single dumbbell or bar and works the whole upper body. And don't let its simplicity fool you!

Stand at one end of a yoga mat or other sturdy surface. Bend over, placing your hands on the mat, getting as close to your feet as you are able (this exercise will also help with your overall flexibility). Use your hands to slowly walk your body out into a plank position, then lower to a push-up, flow into upward dog, back down for another push-up, and then walk yourself back to standing position.

See below for an idea of the movements:

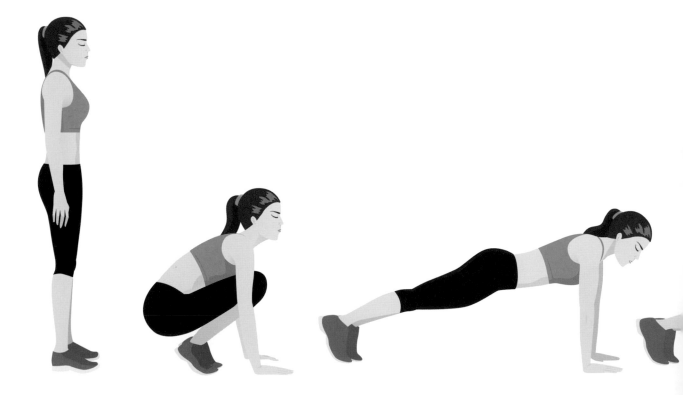

For this 30-day challenge, you'll start with however many walkouts you're able to do. If you can complete the sequence only once, then that, my friend, is where you'll start. If you can do 10 right now, then start there. There is no judgment, just start where you can! Then add one more sequence each day for 30 days.

You'll be amazed by how toned your arms will become doing this every day. And the best part is that you can do this challenge anywhere: home, gym, camping, hotel, etc. So no excuses!

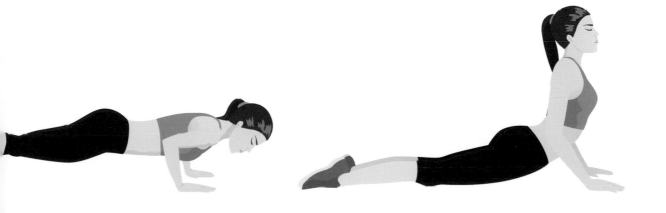

36. DO SIT-UPS AS A FAMILY

Keeping kids active or even interested in being active can seem like a war you wage against the dreaded screens. I'm pretty sure I'm not the only parent that struggles with getting their kids active and cutting back on screen time.

One way that has worked to support more activity in our home is challenges like this one, and sit-ups are an easy exercise that most kids can do. The idea is to just get in the habit of moving with your kids every day and make sit-ups a part of your bedtime routine.

Every night as you're all getting ready for bed, complete a set of sit-ups. You can start with five a night and add a few more every week.

Listen to your kids and let them lead the way with how many they can do. Unless, of course, they say they can't do it; in that case, encourage them and let them know they can! Celebrate completing the challenge with a fun game or movie night as a family.

TIP:

» If your kids are struggling, have them tuck their toes under a couch for extra support.

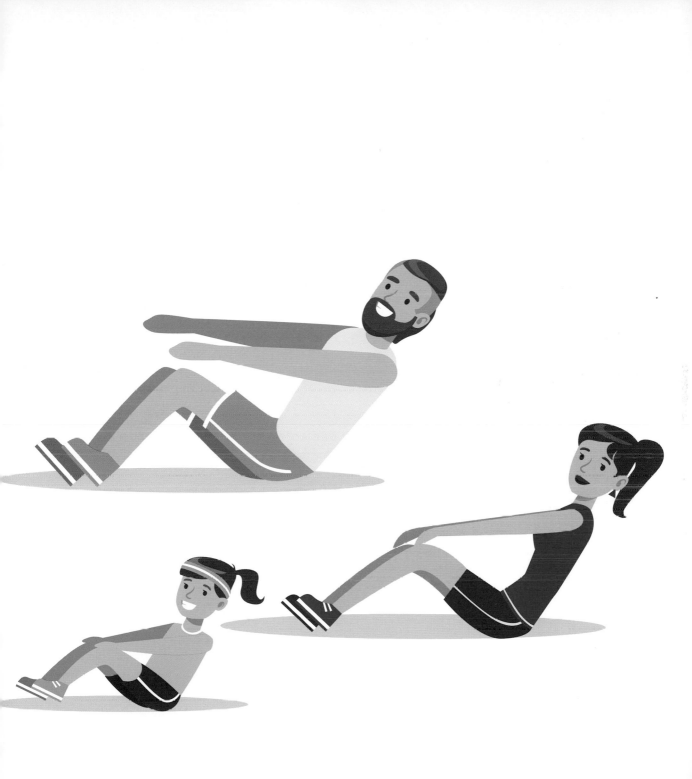

37. BUST YOUR BUTT AND GUT

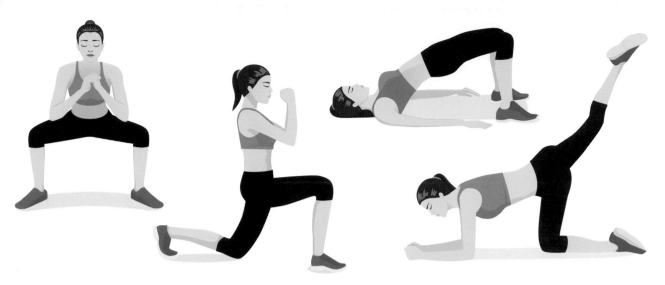

Almost without fail, when I'm talking with women about their bodies, the biggest "problem" areas I hear about are their butts and guts. If you don't know how to do an exercise, go to www.maybeiwill.com/challengesbook for instructions.

So I thought a 30-day challenge completely dedicated to tighter tushes and stronger abs would be a fun one to include. Follow this workout plan for results you can feel in just 1 month:

Day 1:	10 Sumo Squats and 10 Sit-Ups
Day 2:	10 Lunges and 30-second Plank
Day 3:	10 Deadlifts and 15 Ab Leg Lowers
Day 4:	10 Reverse Lunges and 30-second Side Plank (both sides)
Day 5:	15 Plie Squats and 15 Bicycle Crunches
Day 6:	15 Curtsy Lunges and 35-second Plank
Day 7:	Rest
Day 8:	20 Jump Squats and 20 Roll-Ups
Day 9:	15 Glute Bridges and 35-second Plank

Day 10:	20 Donkey Kicks and 25 Sit-Ups
Day 11:	20 Lunges and 40-second Side Plank (both sides)
Day 12:	25 Sumo Squats and 25 Ab Leg Lowers
Day 13:	25 Deadlifts and 25 Bicycle Crunches
Day 14:	Rest
Day 15:	20 Lunges and 45-second Plank
Day 16:	25 Glute Bridges and 15 V-Ups
Day 17:	30 Plie Squats and 25 Sit-Ups
Day 18:	25 Reverse Lunges and 50-second Plank
Day 19:	35 Squats and 25 Ab Leg Lowers
Day 20:	30 Donkey Kicks and 30 Roll-Ups
Day 21:	Rest
Day 22:	25 Deadlifts and 55-second Plank
Day 23:	30 Curtsy Lunges and 15 V-Ups
Day 24:	40 Sumo Squats and 30 Bicycle Crunches
Day 25:	30 Reverse Lunges and 60-second Side Plank (both sides)
Day 26:	30 Glute Bridges and 30 Ab Leg Lowers
Day 27:	45 Squats and 35 Sit-Ups
Day 28:	Rest
Day 29:	35 Lunges and 60-second Plank
Day 30:	50 Sumo Squats and 20 V-Ups

38. BUILD A STRONGER BACK

Having a strong back can not only be sexy, but it can also help us to prevent injury in our everyday lives. We depend on our backs for so much of our day-to-day movements. Whether we are moving boxes, lifting our kids, or even sitting at a desk all day, having a healthy, strong back is essential to living a healthier, happier lifestyle.

As we get older, we are more prone to injury, especially back injury. I'm willing to bet good money that you have had a stiff back just by sleeping or twisting it wrong. While I can't guarantee this will never happen to you again, I can help you to be less prone to these types of injuries.

Doing these exercises for 30 days will help you create a healthier, and dare I say, sexier, back!

If you don't know how to do an exercise, go to www.maybeiwill.com/challengesbook for instructions.

For any exercise performed on both the right and left side of the body, like lunges, do the number of reps indicated on both sides before continuing.

Day 1:
5 Supermans
5 Upright Rows
10 Renegade Rows

Day 2:
5 Supermans
5 Lateral Raises
10 Plank Jacks

Day 3:
5 Supermans
5 Reverse Flys
10 Mountain Climbers

Day 4:
5 Supermans
5 Bent-Over Rows
10 Renegade Rows

Day 5:
5 Supermans
5 Upright Rows
10 Plank Jacks

Day 6:
5 Supermans
5 Lateral Raises
10 Mountain Climbers

Day 7: REST

Day 8:
10 Supermans
10 Reverse Flys
15 Plank Jacks

Day 9:
10 Supermans
10 Bent-Over Rows
15 Renegade Rows

Day 10:
10 Supermans
10 Uprights Rows
15 Mountain Climbers

Day 11:
10 Supermans
10 Lateral Raises
15 Plank Jacks

Day 12:
10 Supermans
10 Reverse Flys
15 Renegade Rows

Day 13:
10 Supermans
10 Bent-Over Rows
15 Mountain Climbers

Day 14: Rest

Day 15:
15 Supermans
15 Upright Rows
20 Plank Jacks

Day 16:
15 Supermans
15 Lateral Raises
20 Renegade Rows

Day 17:
15 Supermans
15 Reverse Flys
20 Mountain Climbers

Day 18:
15 Supermans
15 Bent-Over Rows
20 Plank Jacks

Day 19:
15 Supermans
15 Upright Rows
20 Renegade Rows

Day 20:
15 Supermans
15 Lateral Raises
20 Mountain Climbers

Day 21: REST

Day 22:
20 Supermans
20 Reverse Flys
25 Plank Jacks

Day 23:
20 Supermans
20 Bent-Over Rows
25 Renegade Rows

Day 24:
20 Supermans
20 Upright Rows
25 Mountain Climbers

Day 25:
20 Supermans
20 Lateral Raises
25 Plank Jacks

Day 26:
20 Supermans
20 Reverse Flys
25 Renegade Rows

Day 27:
20 Supermans
20 Bent-Over Rows
25 Mountain Climbers

Day 28: REST

Day 29:
25 Supermans
25 Upright Rows
30 Plank Jacks

Day 30:
25 Supermans
25 Lateral Raises
30 Renegade Rows

39. GET FLEXIBLE

Becoming more flexible is a great way to keep your muscles loose and limber to prevent injury and help you improve your posture, which are big wins in my book!

For this challenge we will focus on stretching for just 5 minutes every day. By taking the time to stretch daily, you'll help your tight muscles relax and, in turn, your muscles will become more flexible and limber, helping you to respond with grace and agility throughout your day. If you don't know how to do an exercise, go to www .maybeiwill.com/challengesbook for instructions.

Here are my favorite exercises for improving flexibility. Choose one to three every day to focus on and you'll be rocking this challenge! Your newly limber body will thank you.

- → **Head Rolls**
- → **Cross-Body Stretch**
- → **Cat/Cow Stretch**
- → **Fold Over Stretch**
- → **Downward Dog**
- → **Reclining Pigeon**
- → **Hip Flexor Stretch**
- → **Hamstring Stretch**
- → **Calf Stretch**
- → **Cobra Stretch**

- → **Standing Triceps Stretch**
- → **Standing Quad Stretch**
- → **Butterfly Stretch**
- → **Scissor Hamstring Stretch**
- → **Single Hamstring Stretch**
- → **Knee-to-Chest Stretch**
- → **Child's Pose**
- → **Lying Knee Twist**
- → **Twisting Glute Stretch**

Every day for 30 days, choose one to three of the above exercises and stretch for 5 to 10 minutes.

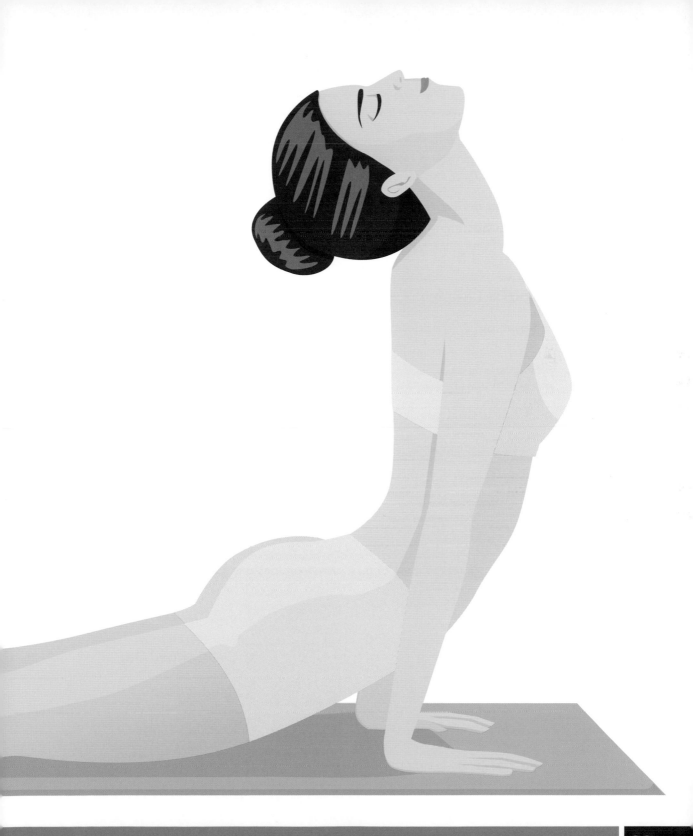

40. PRACTICE YOGA

For this challenge, you'll simply try a new yoga pose every day for 30 days. If you are new to yoga, this is a great way to try it out and realize that yoga is fun and easy to do in any location.

So remove from your mind the images of super-bendy gals doing impossible poses with their abnormally limber bodies. Yoga is for everyone—even you! If you don't know how to do a yoga pose, see page 126. You can also go to www.maybeiwill.com/challengesbook for instructions.

Each day, try the pose a few times to get comfortable with it. Maybe even add on some others that you have previously tried.

Day 1:	Downward Dog	**Day 16:**	Puppy
Day 2:	Warrior 1	**Day 17:**	Bow
Day 3:	Child's Pose	**Day 18:**	Upward Salute
Day 4:	Warrior 2	**Day 19:**	Sphinx
Day 5:	Mountain	**Day 20:**	Seated Forward Fold
Day 6:	Chair	**Day 21:**	Camel
Day 7:	Triangle	**Day 22:**	Boat
Day 8:	Tree	**Day 23:**	Side Plank
Day 9:	Bridge	**Day 24:**	Cat/Cow
Day 10:	Corpse	**Day 25:**	Cobra
Day 11:	Plank	**Day 26:**	Pigeon
Day 12:	Chaturanga	**Day 27:**	One-Legged Dog
Day 13:	Upward Facing Dog	**Day 28:**	Seated Twist
Day 14:	Half Moon	**Day 29:**	Crescent Lunge
Day 15:	Warrior 3	**Day 30:**	Plow

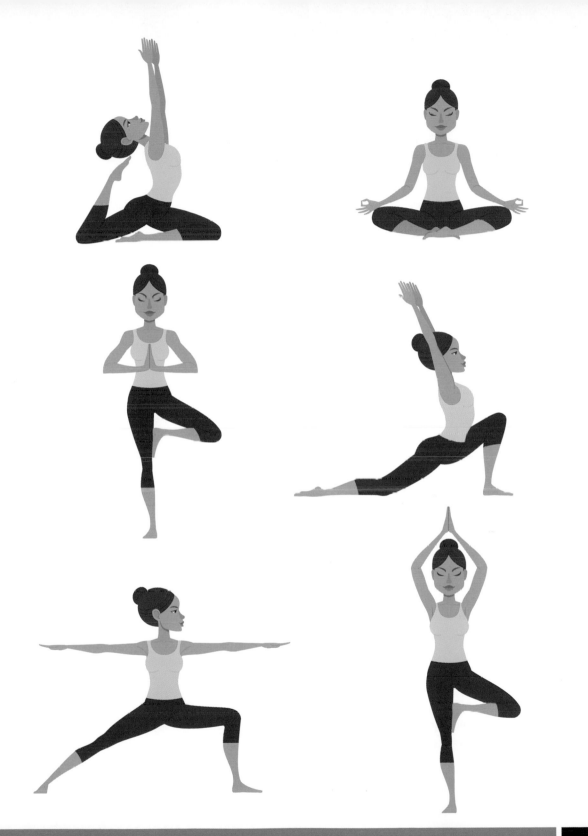

41. DO A FAMILY YOGA CHALLENGE

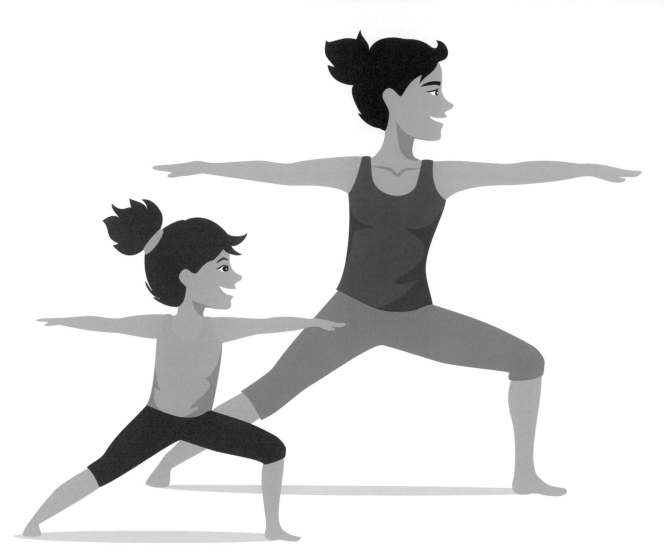

Yoga is an amazing form of exercise to teach your children. It helps children to enhance their flexibility, strength, coordination, and body awareness. It can also help with their concentration, provide a sense of calm, and help them relax.

Doing this yoga challenge as part of your bedtime routine is a great way to help your kids wind down and get ready to go to sleep. Or are my kids the only ones that seem to get more riled up as soon as 8 p.m. hits?

Yoga poses are illustrated on page 126. You can also go to www.maybeiwill.com/challengesbook for instructions on how to do all the poses mentioned in this challenge.

For this challenge, create a "yoga deck" of poses, and every night for 30 days allow your kids to pick five yoga poses to flow through. Parents can get in on the fun too! Yoga is equally beneficial for you, and your kids will love seeing you try to do the poses alongside them.

→ Boat
→ Bridge
→ Butterfly
→ Cactus
→ Cat
→ Chair
→ Child's Pose
→ Cobra
→ Corpse
→ Cow
→ Crow
→ Dancer
→ Dolphin
→ Downward Dog
→ Easy Pose
→ Extended Side Angle
→ Forward Bend
→ Frog
→ Gorilla
→ Half Bow
→ Happy Baby
→ Hero
→ Knee to Chest
→ Legs Up the Wall
→ Lion

→ Locust
→ Lotus
→ Mountain
→ Pigeon
→ Plank
→ Pyramid
→ Reclining Butterfly
→ Runner's Lunge
→ Seated Forward Bend
→ Seated Half Twist
→ Tree

→ Triangle
→ Upward Facing Dog
→ Upward Salute
→ Warrior 1
→ Warrior 2
→ Warrior 3
→ Wheel
→ Wide-Leg Forward Bend

42. FOAM ROLL

If you are new to working out and lifting weights, the challenges in this book will cause you to be sore and you may experience body aches. This is totally normal as you start to build up muscles that have been underutilized. This is where foam rolling can be a fantastic tool to help ease tight muscles and help you to recover faster so you're ready to take on more challenges the next day! In addition, I recommend taking warm baths using Epsom salt and magnesium flakes, two powerhouses when it comes to helping soothe aching muscles.

If you don't know how to do an exercise, go to www.maybeiwill.com/challengesbook for instructions.

Every night before you go to bed for the next 30 days, take 5 to 15 minutes to roll out your aching muscles. You want to roll to a point where you can feel the tension, hold it for a few moments, then release.

Here are some easy exercises you can try if you are new to foam rolling:

1. **Upper Back Roll**
2. **Calf Roll**
3. **Groin Roll**
4. **IT Band Roll**
5. **Hamstring Roll**

6. **Quadricep Roll**
7. **Lats Roll**
8. **Glutes Roll**
9. **Lower Back Roll**
10. **Chest Roll**

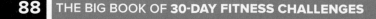

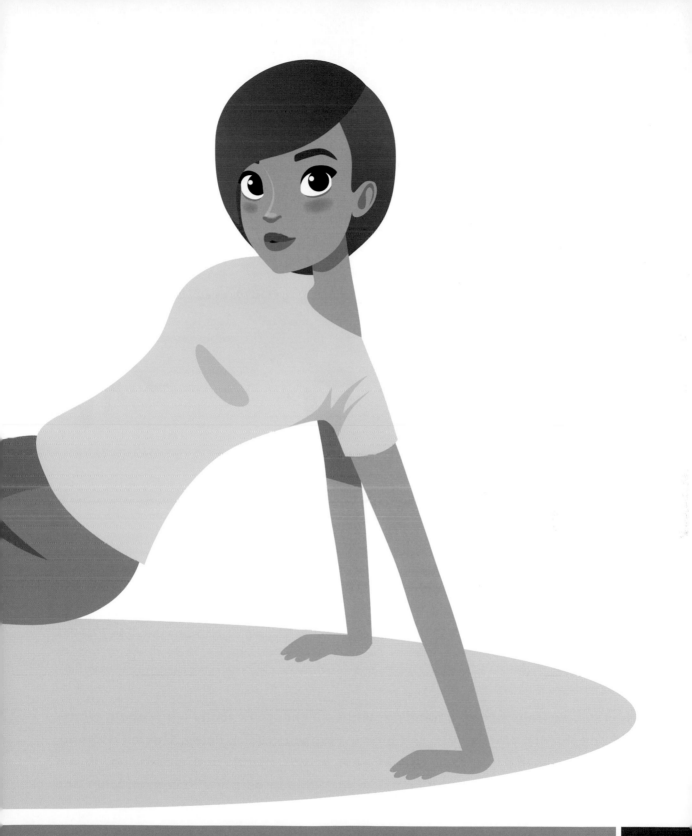

43. SPICE UP YOUR DINNER ROUTINE

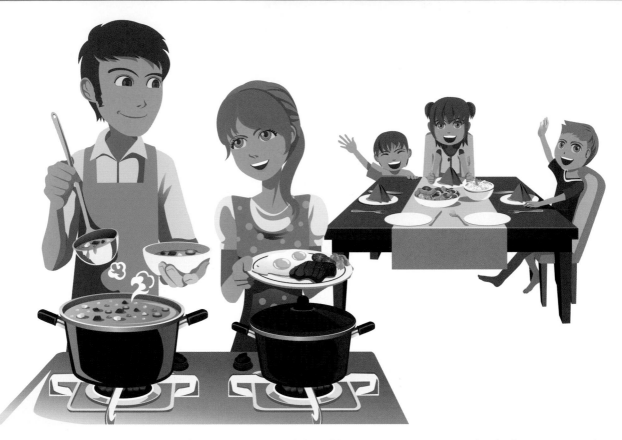

Before I had kids, I envisioned my family sitting around the table, everyone enjoying each other's company and eating a healthy meal together every night of the week. And when my kids were little it was easy, but as they've gotten older, getting us all around the dinner table at the same time can be a major struggle.

I strive to get us all around the table at least three to five times a week. Look over your family's schedule and choose a realistic number of nights that will work for your family. If eating together only two nights a week is all you can do, then that is the number of nights you will use for the challenge: For 30 days, you'll strive to eat together two times a week! If you live solo, try to sit down at a table for dinner those two nights without distractions like your smartphone or television.

When you eat together as a family you have a chance to really learn about what's going on in each other's lives and how everyone is really doing. Having a strong, healthy family life is also a part of your overall health and well-being. In our family we love to play a few games at the table to help invite conversation and

interaction instead of a quick shoveling in of food and an immediate request to be excused.

SWEET AND SOUR

Each family member takes a turn and shares the sweetest part of their day and the sourest part of their day. This provides the kids with an open forum to discuss what may be bothering them, while also reminding them to focus on the positive.

WHAT WE LOVE

Each person takes a turn saying what they love about each family member and also what they love about themselves. We also have a rule you cannot repeat the same things someone else has already said! This is important so that everyone gets to hear more than just "you're nice" a bunch of times.

MIX UP DINNER

Here are some fun ways to breathe new life into the daily routine:

» Choose a country and prepare food from that country.

» Everyone talks with an accent.

» Breakfast for dinner is always a hit!

» Candlelight meal—it's not just for a romantic night in with your partner. Kids love turning down the lights and having a "fancy" meal in the glow of candlelight.

» When the weather is warmer, eat outside and enjoy the evening.

» Potluck night—each child is assigned either a main dish, appetizer, side dish, salad, or dessert. They get to choose what to serve and help make it, and we get to dine on everyone's favorites.

» Mix-up night—write all the dinner courses out on little sheets of paper—salad, drink, side dish, dessert, main dish—and put them in a little bowl. Then take turns picking out pieces of paper to decide the order in which you will eat!

» Go out!—family dinner doesn't mean it has to be at home if you're busy and won't have time to make a home-cooked meal.

44. EAT YOUR VEGGIES

Let's face it, veggies get a bad rap. Whether you never grew out of your aversion to veggies as a five-year-old or are just trying to find creative ways to sneak more into your life, this 30-day challenge is for you.

Here are 30 ways to get more veggies. If you find only a handful that will work for you, stick with those. But I challenge you to get adventurous and try all 30 sneaky methods for getting more glorious veggies into your life. Your body will thank you!

1. **Smoothies:** Throw in a handful of spinach or kale into your morning smoothie.

2. **Omelets:** Tomatoes, spinach, mushrooms, peppers, and onions **are all delicious with eggs.**

3. **Oatmeal:** I love adding pumpkin **to my oats!**

4. **Muffins:** Try throwing carrots, pumpkin, or zucchini into muffins.

5. **Spiralize It:** Zoodles (noodles made from zucchini) are a great swap for pasta.

6. **Juice:** Every week I juice together celery, cucumber, spinach, ginger, lemon, and green apples. The flavor combinations are endless.

7. **Sauce:** If you are making a marinara sauce, add more carrots, tomatoes, mushrooms, onions, winter squash, and peppers. Don't like your sauce chunky? Puree!

8. **Quesadilla:** I love making a quesadilla with feta and spinach then dipping it in hummus.

9. **Dip:** Try making a ranch dip with Greek yogurt to make it healthier.

10. **Pizza:** If you're going to indulge in pizza why not opt for thin crust and load it up with veggies?

11. **Mac and Cheese:** I add pureed butternut squash to my sauce.

12. **Brownies:** Pureed spinach or sweet potato can be easily hidden in that brownie goodness.

13. **Pudding:** Adding avocado to pudding will give it a rich texture and flavor.

14. **Mix-Ins:** There are several brands that now offer powdered greens you can add to drinks.

15. **Casseroles:** There are so many ways to get creative with veggies here. Chicken pot pie? Load it up with veggies!

16. **Puree:** Sweet potato, spinach, and butternut squash all make great purees that can easily be snuck into a lot of dishes without changing the flavor at all. Bake a huge batch and freeze it.

17. **Soup:** Soup is a super-easy way to add a ton of veggies to your life.

18. **Get Creative:** Head to a farmer's market or local grocer and make yourself try a vegetable you've never had before.

19. **Roasted:** This is by far my favorite way to eat veggies. Drizzle a sheet pan of veggies with olive oil, salt, and pepper and roast at 425°F for 15 to 20 minutes.

20. **Fries:** Carrots, zucchini, potatoes, and green beans can all make great baked "fries."

21. **Salad:** Search the internet and try a new recipe that looks like a winner to you.

22. **Hold the Bun:** Lettuce wraps are a super-fresh way to enjoy a hamburger or a sandwich without the heaviness of a bun.

23. **Swap Your Burger:** Opt for a veggie burger.

24. **Grilled Cheese:** Try adding spinach, arugula, tomato, or avocado.

25. **Keep Them Handy:** Often we don't opt for veggies because they aren't as convenient as fruit. Take some time and prepare some sandwich bags with your favorite veggies for easy grabbing.

26. **Sandwiches:** Add cucumbers, tomatoes, sprouts, lettuce, onion, mushrooms, avocado, or peppers.

27. **Find a New Recipe:** Sometimes we can get stuck in a rut and can't seem to think of a way to try vegetables. Just go online and find a new veggie recipe to try!

28. **Cauliflower:** Replace rice with riced cauliflower, or even use it to make a pizza crust or bread sticks.

29. **Veggie Tots:** Zucchini tots are delicious. Look for a recipe online.

30. **Baked Potatoes:** Top with steamed veggies and a little bit of melted cheese.

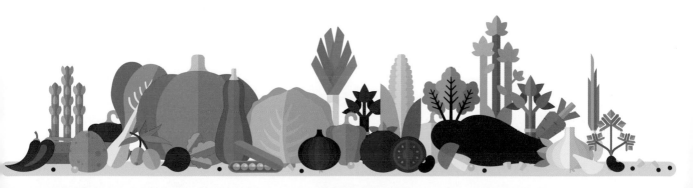

45. DRINK YOUR DANG WATER

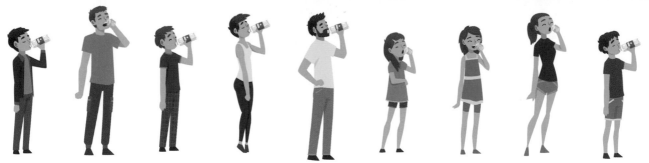

For the next 30 days, challenge yourself to drink a gallon of water a day. Get excited to see what a difference it will make in your overall health and wellness!

Drinking water is a keystone for optimal health and wellness, and I'm a huge proponent of it. But I get the struggle. Trying to get it all in can be exhausting! And let's not get started on the number of trips to the bathroom that are required when one is completely focused on proper hydration.

But luckily, drinking water doesn't have to be dramatic. Like Mary Poppins once said, "In every job that must be done there is an element of fun. Find the fun and *snap!* the job's a game." I am going to show you a fun way to shake up your water consumption and make it a game so you can stay on track and learn to enjoy it.

Learning how to stay on top of your water consumption will help you be healthier and happier to boot. Think of proper water consumption as a major tool in your health and wellness arsenal!

Find a gallon jug and a permanent marker and label it as follows. This will help "visually" keep you on track to meet your consumption goals.

7 A.M. *RISE AND SHINE—I'VE GOT THIS!*
Drink your first glass of water after you wake up to hydrate your body after a long night's rest. This will get your body moving and aide with colon cleansing.

9 A.M. *I'M A ROCKSTAR—KEEP IT UP!*
Drink at least 8 ounces of water 30 minutes before breakfast. This will help your body feel full and improve digestion.

11 A.M. *I CAN DO HARD THINGS!*
Drink at least 8 ounces before lunch.

1 P.M. *KEEP DRINKING! I'M HALFWAY DONE!*

3 P.M. *WATER ROCKS! I FEEL AWESOME!*

5 P.M. *I AM DOING THIS FOR ME!*
Remember to drink at least 8 ounces before dinner!

7 P.M. *NO EXCUSES!*

9 P.M. *TIME TO END THIS LIKE A BOSS!*
Now for the fun part! Infusing your water is a great way to shake things up and amp up the flavor without an ounce of guilt. Here are some delicious, low-calorie additions to help give your water some extra flavor:

→ **Lemon wedges**

→ **Lime wedges**

→ **Blueberries**

→ **Raspberries**

→ **Orange slices**

→ **Strawberry slices**

→ **Kiwi slices**

→ **Mango slices**

→ **Pineapple slices**

→ **Cucumber slices**

→ **Frozen grapes**

→ **Watermelon cubes**

→ **Honeydew melon**

→ **Apple slices**

→ **Mint leaves**

→ **Basil leaves**

→ **Cinnamon sticks**

→ **Rosemary**

→ **Grated ginger**

OR TRY THESE EASY AND DELICIOUS COMBOS:

» Watermelon + rosemary

» Orange slices + strawberry slices + kiwi slices

» Mint leaves + lime slices

» Handful of mixed berries + lemon slices

» Freshly grated ginger + cucumber + lemon slices + mint

» Apple slices + cinnamon sticks

46. TRY GREEN JUICE

Green juice may seem like a passing fad, but I assure you it is not. It's a fantastic way to help you get more nutritious vegetables into your life, especially the "green" ones that are essential for better overall health and wellness. Benefits of green juice include:

→ Power-packed nutrition

→ Provide chlorophyll, which oxygenates your body

→ Improves mental focus

→ Helps boost the immune system

→ Helps aid digestion

→ Reduces inflammation

→ High in antioxidants

→ Helps balance your body's pH levels

With all these benefits it's easy to think grabbing any old green juice is a win, but not all green juices are created equally. Some have tons of added sugars that actually offset any health benefits.

When buying green juices, opt for cold-press green juices. Cold pressing juices helps to protect nutrients during processing. Choose ones that have more veggies than fruit, or skip the hunt altogether and make your own! You can pick up a decent juicer for around $100.

Personally, I love celery juice. According to *The Healthy*, celery is nutrient-rich and a great source of vitamins K and C, manganese, magnesium, calcium, potassium, folate, and vitamin B6, as well as riboflavin. Plus, whole celery has anti-inflammatory properties that promote the health of the gut lining and may help regulate digestion.

For this challenge the premise is super-simple: Just drink a green juice every day for 30 days.

AS A REMINDER:

» If buying store bought choose cold-press green juices with more greens than fruit.

» Celery juice is an easy way to complete this challenge.

» There are so many really great dry green juice powders that will work for this challenge as well. Stick with ones that are high in nutrients and low in sugar.

» Make my Feel-Good Green Juice recipe!

FEEL-GOOD GREEN JUICE

2 stalks celery

2 cucumbers

1 (16-ounce) bag spinach or kale

2 knobs ginger

2 lemons

3 green apples

Juice all and combine in one large pitcher or bottle. Drink 8 to 10 ounces daily.

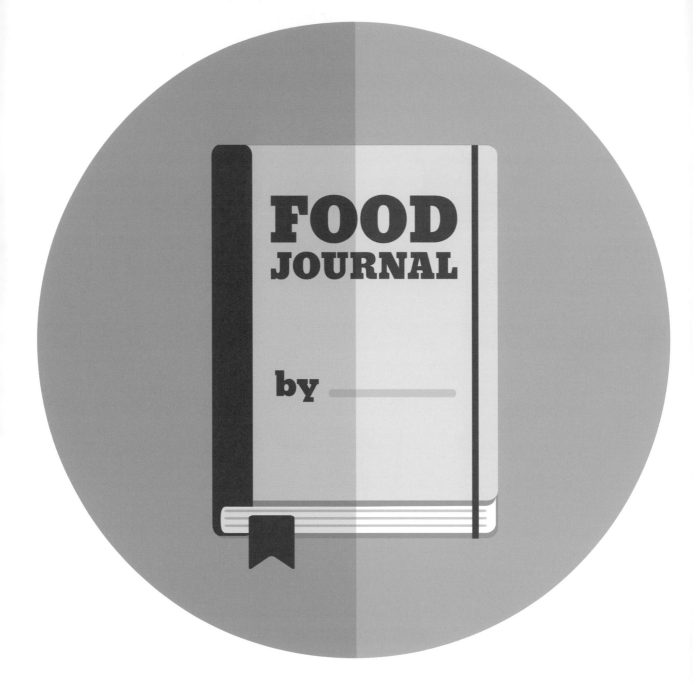

So many times we just eat all day long without any thought as to what we're eating and how we are feeling as we eat. And as we look back at the end of our day, we have no memory of what or how much we actually ate.

I have food journaled off and on for years. Whenever I feel like my eating has derailed and is out of control or my diet starts to resemble that of an unsupervised child at a birthday party, I know it's time to get back to basics and food journal!

Food journaling is super simple. You can use an app like My Fitness Pal or just grab a notebook and a pen. I prefer the pen and paper approach. For me, food journaling is not about logging calories or balancing macros; it's more about connecting my mind to my feelings and recording what I ate as a way to review my progress.

For each meal (even snacks) throughout this 30-day challenge, record the following items:

1. **Level of hunger when you ate, on a scale of 1 to 10, with 1 being not hungry and 10 being starving.**

2. **What you ate. Try and be very specific here and include the amounts eaten.**

3. **How you felt. Where you tired, anxious, bored, happy, or depressed? Tap into the emotional reasons for why you ate. Connecting your emotions to your food choices and food behaviors is super powerful—this is an area you want to really get curious with.**

4. **The time you ate.**

As you look over your data, get curious and review it as you would scientific data. You'll start to see trends emerge. For instance, you might see that everyday around 3 p.m., you eat something unhealthy because you are bored or tired.

Have patience with yourself, be honest, and get curious! Knowledge is power, and this is a great way to objectively see what bad habits you have formed so you can make some changes to help improve your overall health and wellness.

48. TRY INTERMITTENT FASTING

Intermittent fasting is not a diet. It's simply a pattern of eating that has many proven health benefits, including:

ELEVATED HUMAN GROWTH HORMONE: Increased HGH has shown to help with fat loss and muscle gain, both wins in my book.

INSULIN: Insulin sensitivity in some studies showed improvement when people intermittently fasted, where levels of insulin dropped dramatically. Lower insulin levels make stored body fat more accessible to burn as fuel.

CELLULAR REPAIR: When fasting, your cells initiate cellular repair processes. This includes autophagy, where cells digest and remove old and dysfunctional proteins that build up inside cells.

GENE EXPRESSION: There are changes in the function of genes related to longevity and protection against disease.

Here are three ways you can experiment with intermittent fasting throughout the 30-day challenge.

THE 16/8 METHOD: Also called the Leangains protocol, this involves skipping breakfast and restricting your daily eating period to 8 hours, such as 1 p.m. to 9 p.m. Then you fast for 16 hours in between. For me personally, this is the easiest to adhere to. I stop eating at 7 p.m. and start eating in the morning around 11 a.m.

EAT-STOP-EAT: This involves fasting for 24 hours once or twice a week. For example, by not eating from dinner one day until dinner the next day.

THE 5:2 DIET: With this method you consume only 500 to 600 calories on two non-consecutive days of the week, but eat normally the other five days.

Water, tea, and coffee are all okay to eat while you fast. Do not add sugar! Small amounts of cream or milk are okay. I also recommend a branch-chain amino acid powder dissolved in water while you are fasting. Find one that is less than 20 calories per serving!

Ease yourself into this challenge. The good news is you'll be sleeping for a large portion of your fast, which helps. Here's an example fasting schedule:

Days 1–5:	Fast for 10 hours, between 8 p.m. and 6 a.m.
Days 6–10:	Fast for 12 hours, between 8 p.m. and 8 a.m.
Days 11–14:	Fast for 14 hours, between 8 p.m. and 10 a.m.
Day 15 and beyond:	Fast for 16 hours, between 8 p.m. and 12 p.m.

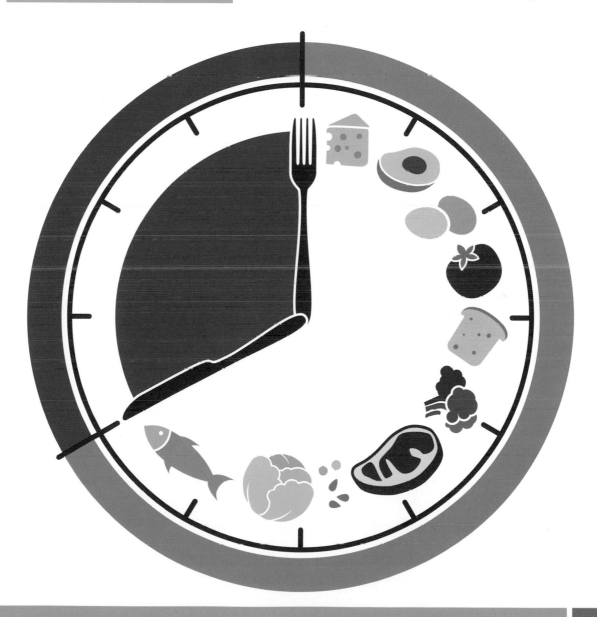

49. KEEP A GRATITUDE JOURNAL

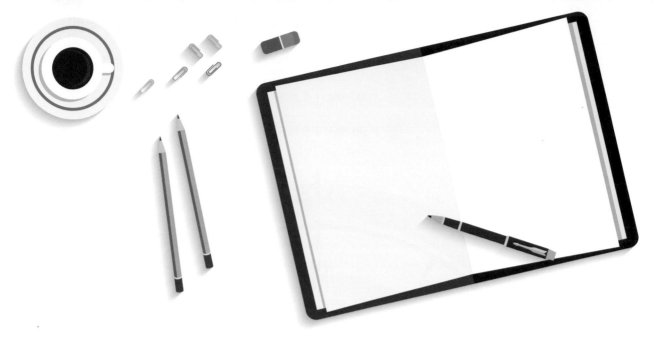

Friends, we are blessed with so much every day! The secret to happiness is recognizing and showing gratitude for those ever-present blessings.

During this 30-day challenge, every night before you go to bed take 5 to 10 minutes and write 10 things that you are grateful for. It can be as simple as that you are alive and your lungs are breathing, that you hit every green light on your way home, that you scored an amazing parking space, that a neighbor just happened to show up when you needed some real help. If you pay attention, you will notice countless little synchronicities that are showing up for you every day. Wake up, take note and express sincere gratitude for it all. Your happiness will increase exponentially.

If you are still struggling on what to write in this little gratitude journal of yours, here are 30 prompts to help inspire you:

1.   **Write about a friend who is always there for you.**
2.   **Write about a favorite (or former) pet that has meant a lot to you.**
3.   **What's a mistake that you made that now, looking back, led to a positive change?**
4.   **What's a family tradition that you are grateful for?**
5.   **Write about a book you love and how it has inspired you.**
6.   **Write about your favorite part of your home.**

7. Write about your favorite food.

8. Write about something you have recently purchased that you love.

9. Write about what your kids, pets, or friends did today to make you smile.

10. Write about your favorite smell.

11. Write about your favorite childhood toy.

12. Write about a time you felt close to God.

13. Write about a time you felt especially loved.

14. Write about your favorite day.

15. Write about something you accomplished that made you proud.

16. Write about your favorite flower.

17. Write about your favorite season.

18. Write about your favorite TV show.

19. Write about something you love to do.

20. Write about a favorite vacation memory.

21. Write about something that made you feel extremely lucky.

22. Write about your weirdest talent.

23. Write about your favorite kind of weather.

24. Write about what body part or organ you are most grateful for today (like your eyes, lungs, arms, legs, etc.).

25. Write about a time you felt peace.

26. Write about an insect that inspires you.

27. Write about the best piece of advice you have ever received.

28. Write about a favorite gift you have received.

29. Write about the smallest thing you can think of to be grateful for.

30. Write about a time someone was kind to you.

Gratitude is the healthiest of all human emotions. The more you express gratitude for what you have, the more likely you will have even more to express gratitude for.

—Zig Ziglar

50. MEDITATE

Meditation is a crucial instrument to harness the power of thought and cultivate more peace, clarity, and happiness in our lives. Learning to train your brain and focus your attention is essential to thriving and will increase your feelings of empowerment and overall well-being. It will help calm and focus you, and therefore help you reach your goals.

Often if I am feeling stressed, I find myself reaching for food even when I'm not hungry. Instead I take a minute or two and find a quiet spot to meditate. This helps me to calm down and deal with my feelings rather than eat them.

When I meditate I can shut down what often feels like a huge, loud party in my brain and just be. In this space of calm and quiet I can get real inspiration and guidance on how to make changes in my life. Some of my best blog posts and business ideas have come to me via a meditation session. There is a reason most CEOs meditate!

I know at first it can feel very strange to sit in absolute quiet and do nothing. But that is why it is called a meditation *practice*. The more times you practice, the more natural it will feel and become.

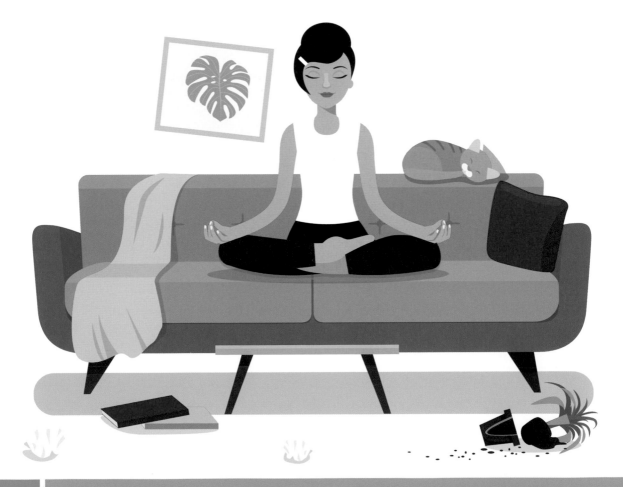

HOW TO MEDITATE

To begin the meditation, sit comfortably in your chair with your shoulders relaxed and spine tall. Place your hands mindfully on your lap, close your eyes, and as much as possible eliminate any stimuli that may distract you. Watch your breath. Simply notice your breath flowing in and flowing out. Don't try to change it in any way. Just notice. Silently repeat a simple mantra, like, "Breathing in. Breathing out." As your mind begins to wander, draw it back to your breath. Notice that as your breath begins to lengthen and fill your body, your mind begins to calm. Consistency is key.

For this 30-day challenge, meditate for 5 minutes first thing in the morning and/or at night. Every day add a minute or two until you are at a good 20 to 30 minutes every day.

Be consistent with your meditation practice, particularly if it is difficult to sit still as you begin. Shorter meditation sessions on a daily basis are more productive than long sessions every few days.

HELPFUL APPS FOR GUIDED MEDITATION

If you're not quite sure how to start meditating, try downloading an app. Many are free or offer paid upgraded versions. My personal favorites are:

» Calm by calm.com

» Simply Being by Meditation Oasis

» Headspace

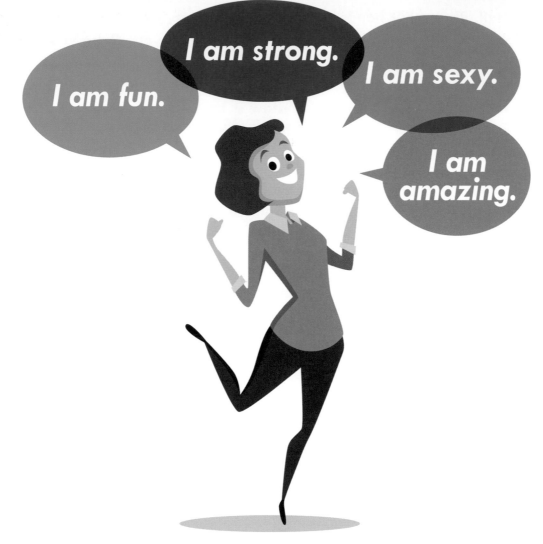

Affirmations, when you first start doing them, will feel slightly ridiculous. Saying these things out loud or even just in your head is going to make you feel like a crazy person. Trust me, I've been there! But I began to become more confident as, day by day, they became more than just words I repeated—they became my truth and each day I began to believe more and more what I was telling myself!

We are the single most influential person in our own lives. If we are repeating to ourselves day after day that we are fat or tired or hideous or worthless, then our mind and body accept that as our truth! Scary!

But would you ever in a million years tell someone else those mean things? Of course not!

So I want you to become your biggest cheerleader, constantly feeding your thoughts with positivity and love. You deserve to love every bit of yourself!

For this challenge I want you to make 30 index cards each with a different "I am" statement. For the next 30 days I want you to read these cards at least every morning and every night. Bonus points if you read them throughout your day. These notecards will be your new best friends. They will be by your side every day for the next 30 days and hopefully always?

Here are some ideas in case you need some inspiration:

→ I am fun.

→ I am *stronger* than any excuse.

→ I am amazing and capable of anything!

→ I am focused.

→ I am perfectly imperfect.

→ I am strong.

→ I am focused and dedicated to making my health a priority.

→ I am worth it!

→ I am a better version of myself every day!

→ I am excited to take care of my body.

→ I am loved.

→ I am an awesome _____ (friend, wife, mother, father, coworker).

→ I am happy.

→ I am filled with joy.

→ I am grateful.

→ I am patient.

→ I am healthy.

→ I am smart.

→ I am confident.

→ I am good at making money.

→ I am lovely.

→ I am sexy.

→ I am good at what I do.

→ I am a good friend.

→ I am blessed.

→ I am unique.

→ I am the best me.

→ I am a rock star.

→ I am amazing.

→ I am grateful to be me.

→ I am in love with who I am.

Not all of these will speak to you, and there might be other things you need or want to focus on. Just know there is downright magic when we place the words "I am" before anything, so be very careful with what you put after those two words.

52. PRACTICE SELF-LOVE

I want you to look in the mirror for a few minutes. What do you see? Are you picking apart the person staring back at you? Do you hate who you see? Do you love who you see? Think about the emotions you feel when you honestly see yourself.

Why are we so hard on ourselves? Learning to love ourselves "as is" is hard! But learning to accept ourselves and embrace and love even the things we hate is so important. By being confident in our own skin and honestly loving ourselves we'll become better spouses, parents, friends, siblings, aunts and uncles, sons and daughters! When we learn to love and accept our body, it helps us to make fitness and health a priority because we love ourselves enough to take care of our bodies and recognize them as the gift that they are.

I used to hate looking in the mirror. I hated seeing that doughy, homely, fat lady staring back at me every morning. I would stare at the mirror criticizing and picking myself to death. My nose was too big, I had too many freckles, my legs look like tree stumps, and my butt was too big... the list went on and on. Finally as I started to be brave, I chose to stare down that woman in the mirror and I told her to *stop!*

I started small by beginning to find small things I liked about myself. I am a good mom. I am a good wife. I like my green eyes. Little by little, I began to believe myself. I began to realize that although my butt might be big, it was my butt. And guess what? I like having a little junk in my trunk. My tree stump legs are crazy strong and enable me to run long distances and power up tall mountains. My freckles are unique and make me who I am.

By staring yourself down and looking at the things you hate and then forcing yourself to find something you like about those same things, you will start to learn to love and appreciate yourself.

So for this self-love challenge, every day for 30 days I want you to pick a body part or a characteristic you dislike about yourself, then flip it and write down five reason why you should *love* it.

For example, I hate my big nose, but...

1. **I am grateful for my ability to smell.**
2. **It gives my face character.**
3. **I see a piece of my ancestors in me who also have shared our infamous "Cuthbert" nose.**
4. **It allows me to breathe deeply when mediating.**
5. **No one else has a nose exactly like mine. It is unique.**

You get the idea. Take the next 30 days and focus on learning to appreciate and love all the things about yourself that you have written off as disgusting, ugly, or whatever unhelpful adjective of choice you've chosen to use.

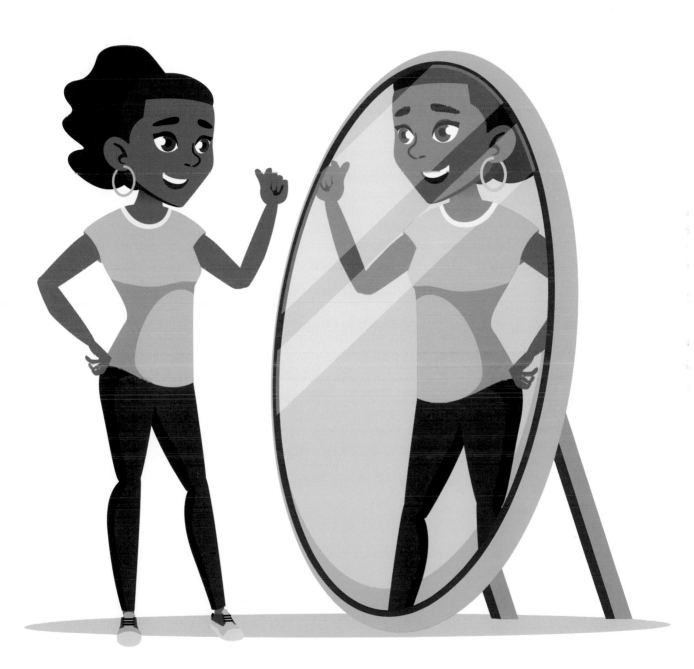

53. PRACTICE VISUALIZATIONS

Humans are very visual beings. We often do not believe something is even possible until we can see it with our own eyes. Plus, our thoughts are extremely powerful, and they ultimately shape our reality. That is why affirmations while using visualizations are very powerful in changing your everyday life.

You can even use visualizations to help you envision yourself as a healthier, happier, more fit version of yourself.

Let's take a step back. Have you ever found yourself thinking about something or someone, and almost like magic that item appears or that person calls or sends you an email? It is pretty amazing how our brains work to create our reality. You can use your powerful thoughts, along with concentration and visualization, to help bring your dreams to life.

Day 1:	Create a vision board—spend some time on this and really think about what you would like your life to look like! I recommend starting small with things you believe can happen for you. For example, "Make an extra X dollars this month." If you put down that you want a million dollars, your brain will likely reject this thought, because you honestly don't believe it's possible.
Days 2–30:	Spend 5 to 10 minutes daily, ideally first thing in the morning and right before bed, focusing on your vision board. Go through each item, focus on it, and allow yourself to visualize having possession of it. How does it feel? The more emotions you can add to your practice the better!

The best part of this challenge is that you are permitted to daydream every day about how you want your life to look and feel. The first time I did this I was dumbfounded by how things started to shift in my life.

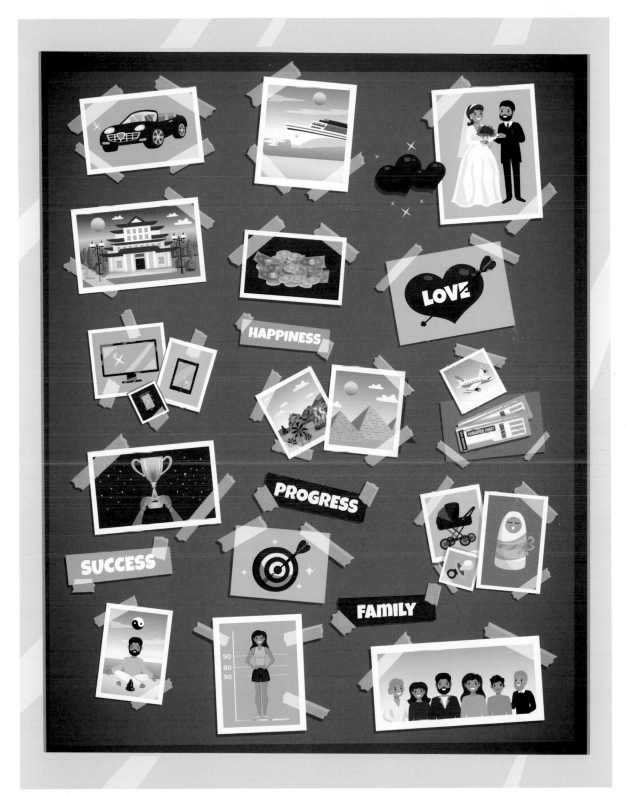

54. SET INTENTIONS

How do you wake up every morning? Do you instantly look at your phone and review texts and emails, allowing others to dictate what your day will look like?

With this challenge, the hardest part will be not to touch your dang phone until you have been quiet and focused on what *you* want your day to look like. Not your boss, not your partner, not your kids, you!

For 30 days, wake up every morning and spend 10 to 15 minutes focusing on what you want your day to look like and what you would like to accomplish! The goal here is to set clear intentions for how you would like your day to go.

When you begin setting clear intentions you begin to take control of your days and retain your own power. Use that power to set the intention to make your own health and wellness a priority!

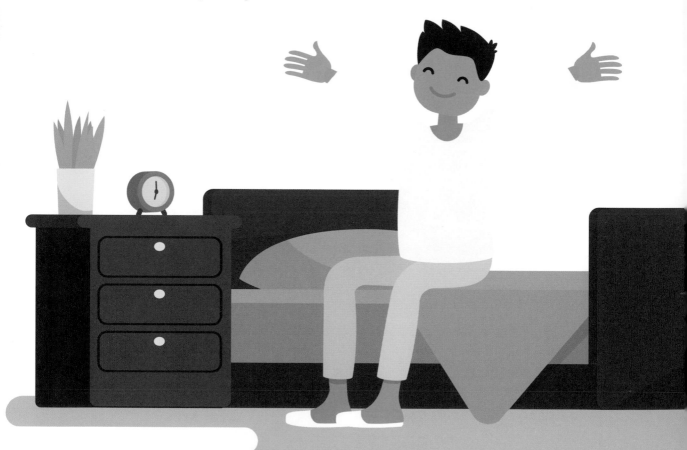

After your alarm goes off, head to a table or comfortable place and pull out your planner or notebook. Allow yourself to be quiet, calm your mind, and ask yourself what absolutely needs to get done today, what you would like to get done today, and what is one thing you can do to help move your needle forward in your personal life, your overall health and wellness, or your business.

Make lists of all your "need to dos," your "like to dos," and your "one thing." Then prioritize and schedule them.

By taking this time before the onslaught of emails and texts come flying in, you can avoid getting lost in the shuffle and losing focus. You can just come back to your lists and know what your priorities are.

Note: This challenge pairs well with the Get Up Early challenge on page 118.

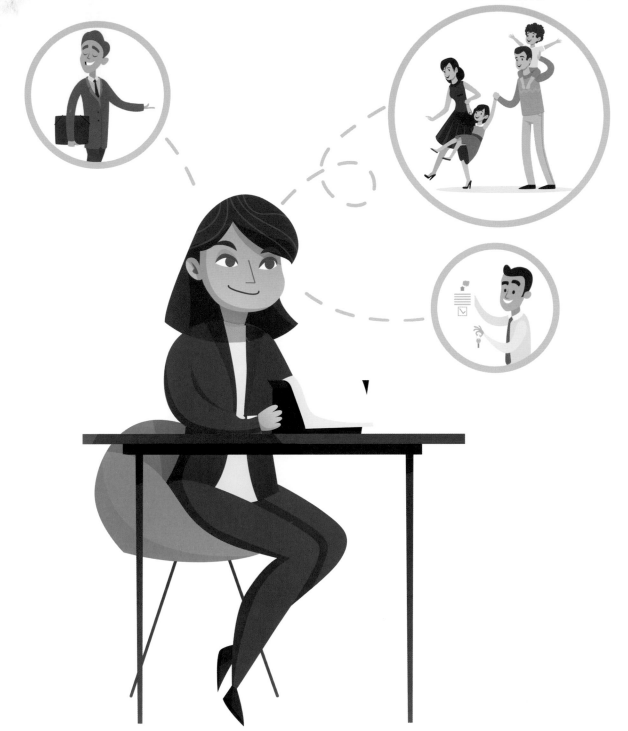

Have you ever sat down and really thought about what you want out of life? Unfortunately most of us focus more on what we don't want in our lives than what we do want. We focus our thoughts on things like fear of losing jobs, not finding love, losing love, and a whole myriad of worries that we let hang over us.

Spend a few minutes every day focusing and defining what you would like your future to look like, answering questions and taking actions to determine what that is. For each area, get clear on what you have, what you want, and two concrete actions you can take toward your goal. Then write a mission statement about how you would like that part of your life to look and feel. It's easiest to break your life down into eight categories:

→ **Intimate Relationships**

→ **Finances**

→ **Life Purpose/Career**

→ **Family**

→ **Health**

→ **Social**

→ **Self-Care**

→ **Material Wants**

Now that you have created clear goals, it would be a great time to move on to the visualizations challenge on page 110.

56. CREATE NEW HABITS

Habits: We all have them, good or bad. But there's good news, because as a fully functioning adult human you have complete power to change yours.

Our brains create pathways that are programmed to respond and act a certain way under certain triggers. For example, every day around 3 p.m. you might start to get tired and need a little break. A signal is fired on the well-worn pathway in your brain signaling to your body to head over to the break room for a soda and a candy bar, resulting in a "reward" in the form of a quick jolt of energy that helps you get over that afternoon slump.

Now, as rational adults, we know that candy bars and soda aren't good for us, but with that well-worn and firmly planted neural pathway in place, making the switch to a healthier alternative is going to take some work!

The first step is to identify the bad behavior or habits you would like to change. Figure out what triggers it. Feeling tired at 3 p.m.? Ask yourself what reward your body thinks it is getting. Identifying the "triggers" for the behavior makes it much easier to change the habit.

On Day 1 of this challenge, you'll make out a list of bad habits or behaviors you want to break.

You will then choose one habit—yep, just one. For this to work you need to focus on one behavior at a time. Of course, you can repeat this challenge until you are able to tackle everything on your list.

Using this method of breaking down habits and identifying triggers is a great way to pinpoint what areas may be holding you back from making your fitness a priority. You can easily use this method to make daily fitness a new daily habit!

Day 1:	List all habits or behaviors you want to change
Day 2:	Pick one and only one to focus on.
Days 3–5:	Observe yourself daily. Take notes on what is triggering your body and mind to respond with the behavior. Get clear on what your triggers are!
Day 6:	Make a game plan! For example, "When my trigger happens, I will do X instead of Y.
Days 7–30	Make the switch. Every time a trigger happens, do the new desired habit. For example, when 3 p.m. rolls around, grab a bottle of water and go for a brisk walk.

Making new healthier habits is so rewarding, but without taking a *real* inventory of your behaviors you are "automatically" looping yourself into patterns that make lasting changes tough. So stick with it! You've got this.

Super curious about the science of habits? Check out these books:

The 5 Second Rule: Transform Your Life, Work, and Confidence with Everyday Courage by Mel Robbins

The Power of Habit: Why We Do What We Do in Life and Business by Charles Duhigg

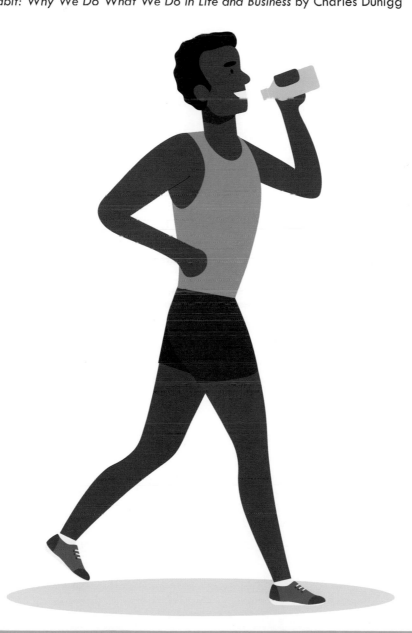

57. GET UP EARLY

After reading the title of this challenge have you already checked out? Getting up early for most people is hard. Nobody wants to spring out of bed, first thing. We all want to linger and stay comfy and cozy in our beds. But when we get up without pushing the snooze button a jillion times, we're taking ownership of our day from the get go!

Not only will you feel more in control of your life but there are so many added benefits to waking up early.

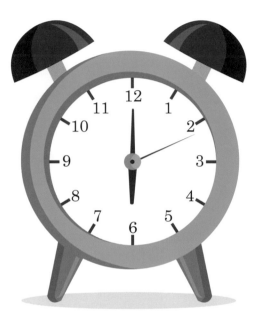

Here's the challenge:

Day 1:	Set your alarm clock 5 minutes earlier	**Day 5:**	Set your alarm clock 10 minutes earlier
Day 2:	Set your alarm clock 5 minutes earlier	**Day 6:**	Set your alarm clock 10 minutes earlier
Day 3:	Set your alarm clock 5 minutes earlier	**Day 7:**	Set your alarm clock 15 minutes earlier
Day 4:	Set your alarm clock 10 minutes earlier	**Day 8:**	Set your alarm clock 15 minutes earlier

Day 9:	Set your alarm clock 15 minutes earlier	**Day 20:**	Set your alarm clock 35 minutes earlier
Day 10:	Set your alarm clock 20 minutes earlier	**Day 21:**	Set your alarm clock 35 minutes earlier
Day 11:	Set your alarm clock 20 minutes earlier	**Day 22:**	Set your alarm clock 40 minutes earlier
Day 12:	Set your alarm clock 20 minutes earlier	**Day 23:**	Set your alarm clock 40 minutes earlier
Day 13:	Set your alarm clock 25 minutes earlier	**Day 24:**	Set your alarm clock 40 minutes earlier
Day 14:	Set your alarm clock 25 minutes earlier	**Day 25:**	Set your alarm clock 45 minutes earlier
Day 15:	Set your alarm clock 25 minutes earlier	**Day 26:**	Set your alarm clock 45 minutes earlier
Day 16:	Set your alarm clock 30 minutes earlier	**Day 27:**	Set your alarm clock 45 minutes earlier
Day 17:	Set your alarm clock 30 minutes earlier	**Day 28:**	Set your alarm clock 60 minutes earlier
Day 18:	Set your alarm clock 30 minutes earlier	**Day 29:**	Set your alarm clock 60 minutes earlier
Day 19:	Set your alarm clock 35 minutes earlier	**Day 30:**	Set your alarm clock 60 minutes earlier

By the end of this challenge you will be gifted with an additional hour every day! Just think how much more you can tackle in that time. You could read, meditate, work out, journal, make a to-do list, or enjoy a little quiet time before your family gets up. But try to *not*: check email or scroll through social media. This is your time, so use it wisely.

When you wake up with intention and spend time first thing giving your day direction you will be amazed by the small or even big changes that happen for you.

58. GO TO BED EARLY

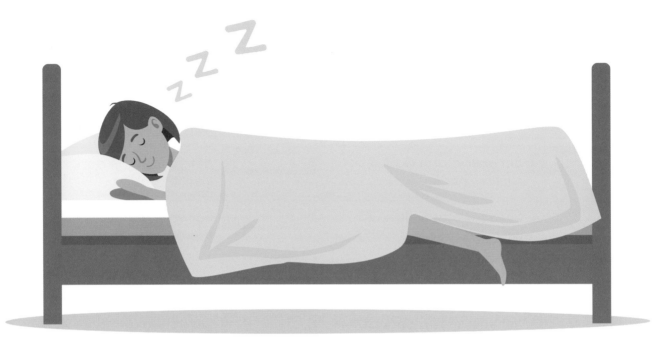

You may or may not have already completed the Get Up Early challenge on page 118, but now the other side of that coin is to get your booty to bed at a decent hour. As they say, early to bed early to rise makes a man (or woman) healthy, wealthy, and wise! And who doesn't want all those things?

On average, a healthy adult needs 7 to 9 hours of sleep. Most of us know our bodies pretty well and how much sleep we really need to function at our best. For example, I do great with 7 hours, whereas my husband needs 9. All of us are different, so listen to your body.

Once you've have thought about how much sleep you need, it's time to calculate a bedtime. So if you need to wake up at 6 a.m. to get ready for work and you know you function best on 8 hours of sleep, then your goal bedtime is 10 p.m.

For the next 30 days, stick to your bedtime! Our bodies thrive on routine and schedules, so try to keep it up even on weekends. And if you sleep in a bit, those are some bonus sleep hours!

Some tips for going to bed on time:

→ Set an alarm on your phone for when you need to get ready for bed.

→ Turn off screens/gadgets 45 minutes before bed.

→ Meditate.

→ Read.

→ Avoid caffeine 6 hours before bedtime.

→ Infuse lavender or lemongrass essential oils in your room to help you relax.

→ Invest in a white noise machine or app for your phone.

→ Try completing the Keep a Gratitude Journal challenge on page 102.

→ Try the Family Yoga Challenge on page 86.

Still on the fence about making your sleep a priority? Did you know sleep plays a huge role in your overall health and wellness? According to the Harvard Sleep Study, sleep deprivation has been linked to the following health issues:

→ Obesity

→ Diabetes

→ Heart disease and hypertension

→ Mood disorders

→ Immune function

→ Decreased life expectancy

→ Stroke

→ High blood pressure

→ Decreased libido

→ Advanced aging

→ Brain fog

→ Impaired judgment

→ Increased risk of accidents

59. CLEAR THE CLUTTER

As a mom of three, I'm quite familiar with clutter. Stuff has a way of expanding and taking up space in our lives. Usually when the clutter situation gets out of control, I start to feel out of control and overwhelmed as well. Even when deadlines loom, I know that if I take the time to clean and tidy up, my energy and focus will improve as well.

Grab some garbage bags and boxes (for donations to charity) and let's get to work.

Day 1: Clean out DVDs and CDs your family no longer watches or listens to.

Day 2: Get rid of free promo T-shirts you do not wear.

Day 3: Throw away the stack of socks without matches.

Day 4: Get rid of your plastic food containers without a matching lid or tub.

Day 5: Clean out your closet. If it does not fit you or you can't remember the last time you wore it, let it go.

Day 6: Clean out your coat closet. Also get rid of mismatched gloves or other oddball items that seem to have landed in this space.

Day 7: Throw away any chipped mugs, plates, and cups in your cupboards.

Day 8: Get rid of all expired medications. Contact your local pharmacy for information on proper disposal.

Day 9: Get rid of old magazines, coloring books, and catalogs.

Day 10: Get rid of extra cords if you have no idea what they belong.

Day 11: Get rid of old greeting cards.

Day 12: Clean out your personal care items, getting rid of things that are expired or that you do not use.

Day 13: Tackle the junk drawer.

Day 14: Get rid of any worn-out underwear.

Day 15: Donate books you no longer read or the kids have outgrown.

Day 16: Clean out your car.

Day 17: Get rid of any expired or stale food in the pantry.

Day 18: Get rid of any expired or "gross" food in your fridge.

Day 19: Go through your paper stacks and get rid of any excess papers and documents.

Day 20: Get rid of kitchen gadgets you never use.

Day 21: Get rid of any worn-out shoes or those you no longer like.

Day 22: Remove unused apps from your phone.

Day 23: Clean out your freezer.

Day 24: Tackle another closet or junk drawer.

Day 25: Clean out your purse and/or wallet.

Day 26: Organize your cleaning supplies.

Day 27: Organize your kitchen cabinets.

Day 28: Organize your office/workspace.

Day 29: Organize and clean up your bedroom.

Day 30: Clean out your linen closet. Get rid of worn-out towels and sheets.

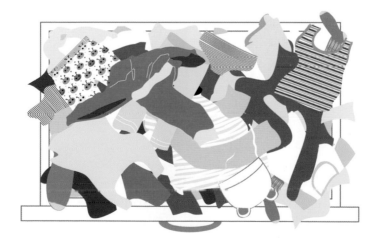

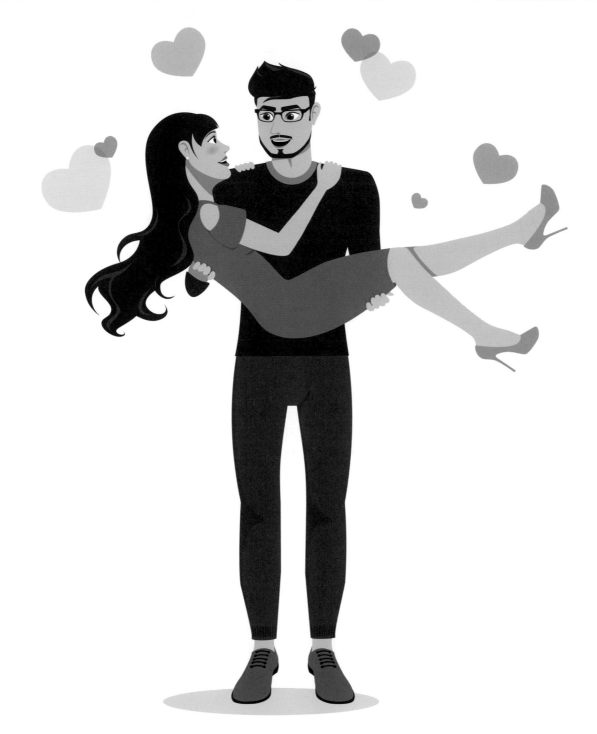

I debated and debated about including this challenge. But I want to share a story with you, because after all these challenges, we're friends, right?

Several months ago, our little family went through a major challenge. My relationship with my husband took a serious toll in the process. We were both dealing with a lot of pain and fear, but in different ways. Instead of pulling together, we found ourselves arguing, fighting, and pulling away from each other. My husband and I have been married for 18 years, and most of them have been extremely happy.

But there we were with this ocean between us that I wasn't quite sure how to fix.

In the midst of this situation, a friend told me about a challenge that completely revamped her marriage. I knew we needed to do something but I wasn't sure what, so I listened with eagerness as to what she was going to say.

As she told me what the challenge was, I was immediately *not* interested. Sex every day?! Are you kidding me? I'm exhausted at the end of the day, and that's the last thing on my mind. With my eyes internally rolling I thought, really, that's what "saved" your marriage? I politely smiled, thanked her for the tip, and immediately thought, nope, not for me.

That night as I lay in bed completely tired and absolutely not in the mood, my friend's words came back to me like a ton of bricks, and I knew that this was something I had to at least try. So I rolled over, pushing away my anger, hurt, and exhaustion and started making a move on my man. I really didn't want to, but I did it anyway.

The next night rolled around and the next night and the next, and little by little I really started to enjoy our sessions. Just like my friend had promised, our marriage started to improve. My happy husband was back, and I felt more loved and secure in our relationship.

So if your marriage is struggling and you have lost that closeness, or you are totally good and just want to amp things up, then this challenge is for you!

The premise is pretty simple: Make love to your partner every night for 30 days. Like me, you may not even be in the "mood," but 3 or 4 days in and your libido and desire will increase.

According to Sandee LaMotte in "10 Benefits of Having More Sex," sex is not just a tool to help improve your relationship, but it's also scientifically proven to help improve your overall health.

→ **Relieves stress**

→ **Improves mood**

→ **Improves sleep quality**

→ **Boosts immune system**

→ **Reduces prostate cancer risk**

→ **Improves cardiovascular health**

→ **Enhances intimacy**

→ **Boosts immune system**

→ **Boosts cognition**

→ **Helps relieve pain**

→ **Burns calories**

APPENDIX

Here are some illustrated yoga poses. Go to www.maybeiwill.com/challengesbook for instructions on how to do all the yoga poses mentioned in this book.

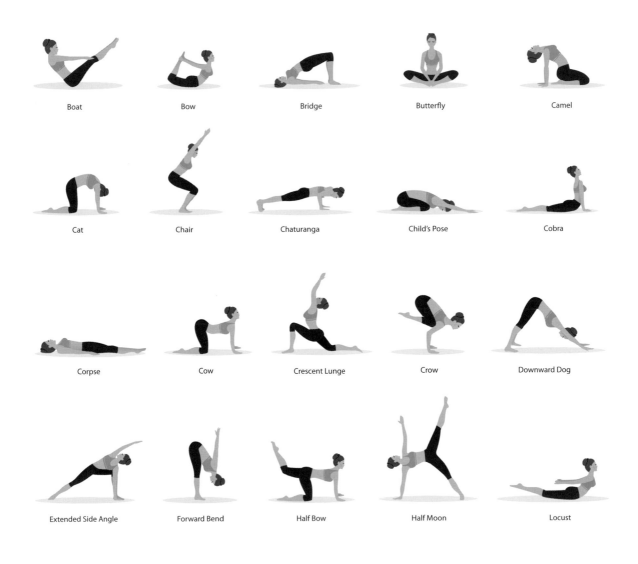

Boat	Bow	Bridge	Butterfly	Camel
Cat	Chair	Chaturanga	Child's Pose	Cobra
Corpse	Cow	Crescent Lunge	Crow	Downward Dog
Extended Side Angle	Forward Bend	Half Bow	Half Moon	Locust

Lotus

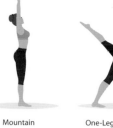

Mountain

One-Legged Downward Dog

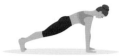

Pigeon

Plank

Plow

Puppy

Pyramid

Revolved Chair

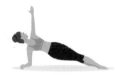

Revolved Side Angle

Runner's Lunge

Seated Twist

Seated Forward Bend

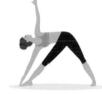

Seated Half Twist

Side Plank

Sphinx

Supine Twist

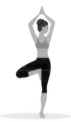

Tree

Triangle

Upward Facing Dog

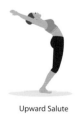

Upward Salute

Warrior 1

Warrior 2

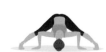

Warrior 3

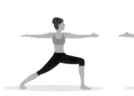

Wide-Legged Forward Bend

ABOUT THE AUTHOR

Andie Thueson is the owner and creator of *Maybe I Will*, a health and wellness website she started over six years ago. She is dedicated to helping readers learn how to live a healthier, happier, and more positive life.

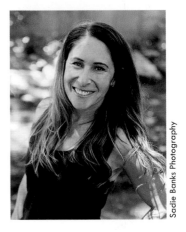

Sadie Banks Photography

Andie knows from experience how hard it can be to stay fit and healthy while raising children or meeting the demands of a career. Her aim is to make fitness and healthy eating simple and fun! Losing weight or getting in shape doesn't have to be an exhausting chore. Andie believes challenges are a great way to harness the power of each day while making REAL, lasting changes in your life.

Andie lives with her husband, Kelly, their three kids, and two goldfish that will not die in Springville, Utah.

Read more about Andie on her website www.maybeiwill.com or follow her adventures on Instagram @andiethues.